December 20/16

May you find words
+ ideas in this study
which edify and
inspire you, as you
do us.

YOUR
PRIVILEGED POSITION

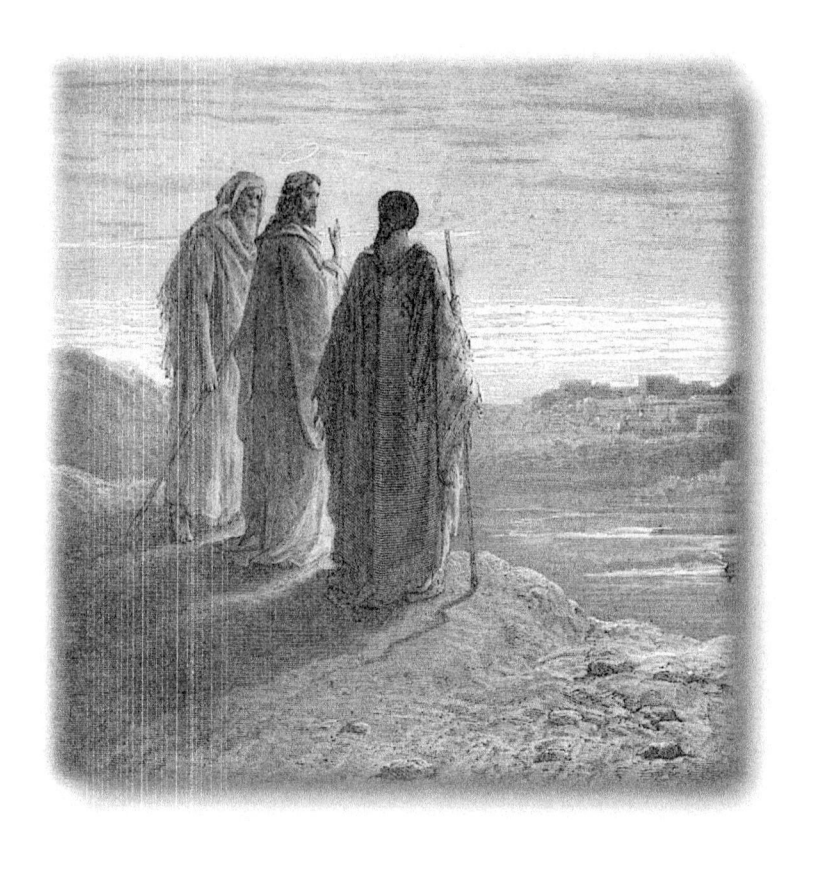

YOUR PRIVILEGED POSITION:

Walking in the Footsteps of Jesus as a Christian in Healthcare

By Paul O. Gerritson, MDiv

Christian Healthcare Insights Publishing
Durham, North Carolina

Copyright © 2016 by Paul O. Gerritson

All rights reserved. No part of this publication may be reproduced, distributed, or transmitted in any form or by any means, including photocopying, recording, or other electronic or mechanical methods, without the prior written permission of the publisher, except in the case of brief quotations embodied in critical reviews and certain other noncommercial uses permitted by copyright law. For permission requests, write to the publisher, addressed "Attention: Permissions Coordinator" at the address below.

Christian Healthcare Insights Publishing
3704 Sunningdale Way
Durham, NC 27707

CHIPublishing@gmail.com

Ordering Information:

Quantity sales. Special discounts are available on quantity purchases by corporations, associations, and others. For details, contact the publisher at the address above.

Printed in the United States of America

First Printing, 2016

ISBN 978-0-9979154-2-6

Cover and Frontispiece Illustration:
Engraving by Gustave Doré
"The Road to Emmaus,"
from *The Doré Bible Gallery,*
(Chicago, Belford-Clarke Co., 1891).
Digitized 2004 by Gutenberg.org.
http://www.gutenberg.org/files/8710/8710-h/8710-h.htm#link092

Editing and Book Design by Margie Tippett

Major headings and text in Palatino
Module headings in Meiryo

Unless otherwise noted, all Scripture quotations are taken from the Holman Christian Standard Bible® 1999, 2000, 2002, 2003, 2009 by Holman Bible Publishers. Used by permission. Holman Christian Standard Bible®, Holman CSB®, and HCSB® are federally registered trademarks of Holman Bible Publishers.

Disclaimer

While the author was an employee of Triangle Christian Medical & Dental Associations (TCMDA) at the time of writing, this communication is not a production of TCMDA. Opinions, technical information, advice, and/or instruction are not necessarily endorsed by TCMDA. While this material is provided as a service, it is without guarantee of results. Implementation of any content found in the communication is done solely at the user's discretion and risk; the author and TCMDA are not responsible for any untoward outcomes. Any mention of political parties, candidates, or legislation relate to commentary on principles and values and do not represent or imply author or TCMDA endorsement of any party, candidate, or legislation.

Dedication

I want to dedicate this book to three godly women who have made indelible marks on my life and this work.

My sister Robin Rodgers was the first Christian I ever actually heard share with boldness what the Lord had done for her and the loving mercy He had had on her. She worked the soil and sowed seeds in me over some 15 years. One day my soil was ready to receive God's offer of abundant life through Jesus and her seeds germinated. Robin has never been rich in any conventional sense, but she continues to show what real abundant life in Christ means.

My late wife Sandy had the ability to see some things in me to which I was blind. Most importantly, she saw God was using all the circumstances of my life to arrive at the place of teaching this material. She made sure I came to see it too.

My new wife Judy loves me unconditionally. That inspires me each and every day to press on, regardless of circumstances or challenges. She exemplifies, in her own unique way, what it is like to walk in the love of God.

May this book take the seeds planted in me by this cloud of witnesses and turn them into a harvest of 30, 60, or 100-fold through you and the lives you will touch after you work through these studies. Amen.

Contents

Dedication vi

Contents vii

Preface viii

Acknowledgments ix

Introduction x

Preliminary Points 1

Format Of This Book 12

Mark 1:1-15 – Prepare the Way: The Messiah is Here! 15

Mark 1:16-45 – The Privileged Position of Christians
in Healthcare 27

Mark 2 – Exploding The Expected Order Of Things 45

Mark 3 – The Irony Of Opposition To Healing Ministry 59

Mark 4:1-34 – Parables Of What Are – And Aren't –
Your Tasks 75

Mark 4:35-5:43 – Tell Of Your Encounter With The
Omnipotent One (Part 1) 91

Mark 6 – Tell Of Your Encounter With The
Omnipotent One (Part 2) 111

Mark 7 – God Knows Our Hearts But Do We? 131

Mark 8 – Spiritual Vision 145

Mark 9 – Christian Healthcare Must Be Bound To Jesus 161

Mark 10 – God's Plan For Healing Relationships 181

Mark 11 – The Double Helix Of Public & Self-Deception ...199

Mark 12 – Small Stories Make For Big Lessons 215

Mark 13 – Labor Pain Principles 235

Mark 14 – Will You Be Found Faithful? 255

Mark 15 – Prepare For Spiritual Warfare 281

Mark 16 – Go Forth In The Promises & Power Of God 299

Appendix I: A Harmony Of The Gospels Outline 312

Preface

Hundreds of healthcare students at UNC Schools of Dentistry, Medicine, and Pharmacy, Duke School of Medicine and Physician Assistant Program, Campbell School of Osteopathic Medicine, and Christian healthcare practitioners of all levels throughout central North Carolina have heard, challenged, and sharpened the material presented in this book.

Credit and gratitude for allowing me to share what I've learned in the form of a study guide must, however, go first to Rory O'Kane, David Crank, Catherine Schricker, and Preston Ford at the UNC School of Dentistry. I'll never forget the cold, dark Tuesday mornings before classes when they asked me to teach them this material in 2013. The looks on their faces and their expressions of gratefulness brought me warmth and light every week. In 2014, Dr. Steve Boyce invited me to bring the material to a Thursday morning Christian practitioner fellowship in Raleigh. As iron sharpens iron, the group's inquiries and comments about the material, rooted as they were in their decades of healthcare experience, were invaluable in inspiring many of the insights and probing questions contained herein.

Acknowledgments

The people who help shape and form us are very special. I want to be sure to acknowledge the wonderful people who invested in me in ways that made this book possible.

Colonel Harold Neal and Lieutenant Colonel Diane Strawn at the 544 Strategic Intelligence Wing, USAF gave me uncommon grace and space to research, test, and prove unconventional concepts. They took big risks on my behalf.

I'm indebted to Larry Cox, my first pastor, for teaching me to see and test all of life against what God's Word says. My second pastor, Dr. Roger Russell, modeled mature faith and devotion to passing it on trustworthily to the next generation.

Dr. Frank Shope at Wayland Baptist University was my first true theological mentor. He constantly challenged me to meditate ever-deeper on the biblical texts to discover what they say. Dr. Darlene Gautsch and Dr. Steve Veteto at Golden Gate Baptist Theological Seminary taught me to study the biblical texts in Hebrew and Greek, respectively, and then write with clarity about what I was discovering.

At Albuquerque Ambulance Service, I first saw Christian healthcare in action watching Barbara Christian, EMT-P. At AAS and Rocky Mountain EMS, Robert Campbell, MIC-P, exemplified excellence, integrity, and humor in healthcare.

Craig Fowler, MD and Amy Fowler, MD are the two most generous people I've ever met. Their hearts for ministering to and transforming Christians in healthcare are seemingly without bounds. I owe them a debt of gratitude for what they've taught me about stewarding God's gifts with joy. The Fowlers also introduced me to Dr. Bill Wilson and his lovely wife Virginia. They became my medical and marital mentors at a time I needed godly people to lift my heavy arms.

Introduction

Shortly after Operation Desert Storm concluded in 1991, my new bride Sandy and I moved to rural New Mexico. There I gave my life to Jesus. She rededicated her life to Him. Together we grew in our faith in the person and work of Jesus Christ.

Simultaneous with becoming a follower of Jesus, I became involved in emergency medical services through the local volunteer fire department. Reading the Gospels and EMS textbooks at the same time, it occurred to me that Jesus used the acts of healing bodies and teaching souls to earn an audience for speaking to people's spirits. I also realized from Gospel reading that Jesus passed that responsibility of healing bodies, teaching souls, and speaking to spirits on to His followers. It seemed a natural fit for me to incorporate healing, teaching, and speaking into my healthcare practice.

It also occurred to me that today, unless God supernaturally gives someone the gift of healing, only Christians involved in healthcare have the capacity to heal, teach, and spiritually speak in a single encounter, as Jesus did. That makes being a Christian and serving others through a healthcare vocation a privileged position! We can walk in His footsteps.

During my career as a 911 paramedic, and then Mobile Intensive Care Paramedic and EMS Operations Director, I took that privileged position seriously. My technical skills, used in conjunction with my faith, were integral to dealing with: sudden shock, suffering, chronic physical and mental illnesses, death, grief, rapid-fire demands for perfection as a technician with no margins for mistakes, long and odd hours, and constant interactions with strangers and peers who didn't always see things the way I did. Healthcare had an inordinate share of stressors.

EMS had joys to be sure. Yet often wrapped in those joys were temptations to think more highly of myself than I ought when things went well. To avoid the trap of hubris, I leaned hard on Jesus. It was the only path to humbly go His way.

God used a bad patient lift to bring my EMS career to a close and move me into vocational ministry. I never stopped believing, though, that Christians in healthcare are *the* people who have the greatest potential to minister. This became all the clearer when Sandy was diagnosed with, and ultimately succumbed to, ovarian cancer in 2012. At the patient end of the stethoscope, we received Christ-like ministry from a very few practitioners. We found ourselves far more often praying for our caregivers and teaching them how to serve in a Christ-like manner. Sandy's last words were encouragement to keep on teaching Christians in healthcare how to walk in Jesus' footsteps. Now God has richly blessed me with my godly, loving wife Judy, who also encourages me to keep ministering to the healthcare community.

To do that, there is tremendous value in going back to the Gospel roots, studying the way of Jesus. While all of God's Word has something to say about living in the image and likeness of God, the Gospel of Mark is the briefest and most straightforward account of how God walked and ministered among us. The teaching of Jesus, the response of the world, and the training of the disciples are clearest and least encumbered. That's why it is the backbone of this study.

May God bless you as you study Mark's Gospel from a Christian healthcare perspective. May you come to see, truly appreciate, and leverage your privileged position.

Paul

Durham, North Carolina, 2016

Preliminary Points

Over the years of practicing healthcare and studying the Gospels, I've come to two conclusions. One is that there is such a thing as "Christian healthcare." It is distinctive and definable. The second is that there are some discernible attitudes and behaviors of Christian healthcare practitioners as well. By the time you finish this book, I believe you'll come to the same conclusions.

Recognizing how very busy Christians in healthcare are, I have chosen to make certain statements based on these two conclusions from the start of the book. To write otherwise and develop the arguments for these conclusions along the way detracts from tightly focusing on Jesus as the archetype of a Christian healthcare practitioner. It would delay your learning to emulate His attitudes and actions. Developing arguments along the way, rather than stating the conclusions up front, can be thought of as grinding eyeglass lenses while the raw glass is on the face of the wearer. Isn't it better for the reader of this study to put on a finished pair of glasses and see well right away? I anticipate the reader will agree on the soundness of this decision and the veracity of the conclusions by the end of *Your Privileged Position*. What follows here, then, are some essential, preliminary points setting the stage for the reader as they delve into the study of Mark's Gospel. I invite you to reflect upon these concepts.

The Biblical Text

> *First of all, you should know this: No prophecy of Scripture comes from one's own interpretation, because no prophecy ever came by the will of man; instead, men spoke from God as they were moved by the Holy Spirit.*
> 2 Peter 1:20-21

All Scripture is inspired [breathed out] *by God and is profitable for teaching, for rebuking, for correcting, for training in righteousness, so that the man of God may be complete, equipped for every good work.*

2 Timothy 3:16-17

For whatever was written in the past was written for our instruction, so that we may have hope through endurance and through the encouragement from the Scriptures.

Romans 15:4

The Holy Spirt somehow moved Mark, and all authors of Scripture, to write what God wanted them to say, using their own voice and vocabulary, grammar, and style. The Gospel of Mark, in its autograph (first written text) was God's chosen breathed-out message to the hearers and readers of Mark's day. Manuscript (subsequent copies of the autograph) evidence and textual criticism makes it abundantly clear that what you have of Mark's Gospel is reliable – including the fact that chapter 16 may not be all Mark's work.

"Whatever was written" is a key phrase. While the exact words you read may change with time and language, the importance of every single word in the autographs should not be underestimated. Each word was given for a purpose – our edification, encouragement, and equipping to do the righteous works of God. Whatever orthodox translation you choose, you are to carefully consider the meaning and purpose of each phrase, clause, or concept. They were preserved by God through two millennia for you to learn from and apply.

You also need to read the texts for their correcting and rebuking, as well as their teaching and training. Many times in this study, the text will seem like a bitter pill that is hard to swallow. Remember though, the pills are for our healing.

Defining Christian Healthcare

In my prior book, *Notes of Encouragement: Reflections on the joy and power of practicing distinctively Christian healthcare*, (Durham, Christian Healthcare Insights, 2016), I presented my definition of Christian healthcare:

> **Exposing** people to Jesus while **excellently** healing bodies, teaching souls, speaking to spirits, and **exuding** the love, wisdom, and power of the Holy Spirit.

This definition has excellent care for the whole person at its core. However, the core is bracketed by two key clauses which distinctively set Christian healthcare apart from any other form of medicine.

The initial clause is the mission statement given to all Christians: Be witnesses of Jesus Christ everywhere you go, including the place you work (See Matthew 28:18-20, Mark 5:18-20, and Acts 1:8). You should not be ashamed to be obedient to God's call on our lives even as you practice our vocation of healthcare. His call is eternal and so infinitely important. Our vocation, no matter how noble, is only temporary.

The closing clause is rooted in two critical facts. To begin with, only a Christian can practice Christian healthcare, for only a Christian is indwelled by God, the Holy Spirit (See 2 Timothy 1:14, 1 Corinthians 3:16, 6:19, and 1 John 3:24). In addition, God the Father and Jesus give every believer the Holy Spirit to equip them with all they need to authenticate the truth of their testimony exposing Jesus (See Galatians 5:22-23, 1 Corinthians 2:1-16, 12:7-8, and Ephesians 3:16).

En toto, the definition of Christian healthcare describes an integrated pattern of thinking and acting as a healthcare practitioner. It describes a sandwich, so to speak, not a loaf of bread, and jars of peanut butter and jelly.

It is one thing to know what Christian healthcare is. It is another to become and remain a Christian healthcare practitioner. Doing so means faithfully and fully serving your Master and those with whom you come in contact. You intentionally do so in general through your healthcare vocation and in particular using your voice. You accept your Christian calling to be His witnesses and ambassadors, striving to act in His power and under His authority. Everything you do and say regarding healthcare, you do according to Jesus' model and with the Holy Spirit's leading.

Jesus often 'purchased' an audience to whom he could speak about the kingdom of God by healing a body and/or teaching a soul with excellence. You are eternally called to be a child and servant of God. Your temporary vocation is healthcare. Your excellent practice of temporarily healing bodies and teaching souls is prerequisite to having a trusting, listening audience when you speak to a person's spirit about eternal matters.

Body, Soul, and Spirit

Jesus' ministry was unique in that He was able in a single encounter to heal bodies, teach souls, and speak to spirits. Let's look just a bit deeper at what these three terms mean, for they will appear over and over again in this study of Mark's Gospel as deliberate actions of Jesus. Jesus tasked His disciples to emulate them.

Heal the Body

The body is the physical, material instrument through which, ideally, the will of the soul is expressed or carried out. The body is not to be thought of as a mere vehicle without intrinsic value, or that the body is somehow 'unclean.' God declared the human body very good – both in word and in the fact Jesus took on human flesh just like ours. God gave the body the ability to appreciate input through the five senses. The body is self-aware, automatically reacting to dangerous or pleasurable stimuli. It is, to an amazing degree, self-repairing and will fight to stay alive.

In the end time, every believer's body will be raised and glorified by God in resurrection, reunited with its soul and spirit. The unbelievers' bodies will be raised too, to a less-than-joyful end. As Christians in healthcare it is important to remember the distinction between resuscitation and resurrection. *Resuscitation* is participating in restoring life to one who appears, according to all signs observed at the time, dead. Resuscitation in no way precludes a future, irreversible, death. You may participate occasionally in a resuscitation. However, God alone performs *resurrection* when He raises, or creates anew from the elements, a tangible, immortal body which is in some way similar to and recognizable as one that had lived. He rejoins the new body to its previously existing soul and spirit.

Healing the body, in the context of this study, doesn't necessarily mean making everything right and whole. This is a broken world and that's not always possible. Healing in this study means striving to enable and empower the body to be as close as possible to what God intended it to be. Then the soul may use it to the maximum extent circumstances permit. Thus it is still a form of healing even if your actions are limited to no more than ameliorating pain or suffering.

Teach the Soul

The human soul is a unique, immeasurable, immaterial aspect of a person. It consists of a person's emotions, intellect, memories, and will. The soul controls the non-autonomic actions of the body. Unlike the body, the soul cannot be cloned. Thus there will never be a duplicate of you. At the creation of mankind, God declared the animated human being to be a "living soul."

In biblical texts, you see that demons, or unclean spirits, can interfere with a soul's capacity to control a body. Casting out an unclean spirit is a manner of restoring the rightful role of an individual's soul to have dominion over its body.

In Romans 12:1-3, you see God's plan for the interaction of soul and body. As the soul is taught new things (is renewed) that should transform how the body is used and cared for. Different choices are made due to learning new things. Different actions and better outcomes should follow.

Speak to the Spirit

The human spirit is also a unique, immeasurable, immaterial aspect of a person. It is the innermost aspect of a person which desires and has the capacity to connect, commune, and walk in agreement with God's Holy Spirit (See Ephesians 3:16). God has put eternity in every person's heart, thus demonstrating each person has a spirit and that He desires every human spirit to know His Holy Spirit (See Ecclesiastes 3:11). It appears that the human spirit is alive and can respond to God *in utero* (e.g., John the Baptist's fetal response in Luke 1:41) but remains in a gestational state until a person believes on the person and work of Jesus, at which time it is "born again" (See John 3:1-21).

The spirit has the ability to unite the natural with the supernatural, including a key role in renewing the soul so that it transforms the actions of the body to say and do things pleasing to God (See 1 Corinthians 2:14-16 and Ephesians 4:22-24). Among those whose human spirit has not been born again, unclean spirits appear to have capacities to control humans by distorting or abusing the things of God. In so doing, they corrupt the thinking of the soul, and thus the words and deeds of the body.

As you have probably already observed, any competent healthcare practitioner can heal a body and teach a soul. Christians don't have a corner on that set of skills. However, Christians do have a corner on being able to speak spiritually about true eternal life, led by the words and prompting of the indwelling Holy Spirit of God. This is called your spiritual voice. Using it as an ambassador and witness, you speak to the spirits of the people around you. Using that spiritual voice will prompt a response in some hearers not unlike that of John the Baptist or the Philippian jailer (Luke 1:39-41 and Acts 16:16-34) – a yearning to trust Jesus and be born again. When you speak with a spiritual voice to those who have already been born again, you can bring hope, comfort, and strength. The ability to speak in a spiritual voice and the potential results are unique to Christians and help define a Christian healthcare practice.

Image and Likeness

> *Then God said, "Let Us make man in Our image, according to Our likeness. They will rule the fish of the sea, the birds of the sky, the livestock, all the earth, and the creatures that crawl on the earth." So God created man in His own image; He created him in the image of God; He created them male and female.*
>
> Genesis 1:26-27

Throughout this study there are references to being created in God's image and likeness. Human beings are the only creations which God specifically declared were created in His image and likeness. While some scholars say 'image' and 'likeness' are synonyms, a careful reading of Genesis 1-2 indicates God created women and men in His image, then walked with them in a personal relationship in order to train, shape, and guide their innate capabilities into His likeness.

God's clearly stated intent was for humans to serve as His regents, His stewards over the earthly creation. Creation should have been able to look at a human being and see the image and likeness of God. However, due to the fall, the image and likeness were and remain marred. As a Christian, you know from God's Word that only through God's work and power can His image and likeness be fully restored – redeemed, regenerated and renewed. For followers of Jesus, restoration occurs progressively, though incompletely, through the sanctification process. Eventually, at the resurrection, perfected restoration will happen instantly, completely, and eternally.

Image – Reflecting God's Greatness

God is great in His character, both in His magnitude and perfection. His greatness includes things like eternal reality, infiniteness, omniscience and omnipotence, spirituality, life, personality, creativity, desire for and constancy in relationships, and the ability to reason facts, consider potential outcomes, and then make choices.

Before the fall, humans created in God's image were intended to reflect God's character – His greatness. All people – regardless of their relationship to God – still reflect to some degree God's greatness. Bearing His image means to have, more or less, the character and nature of God in us. You are neither a god or demi-god. Yet He has put eternity in your heart, and you share with God things like love, an appreciation for community, and a desire for righteousness and justice.

Likeness – Manifesting God's Goodness

God is good and exercises His attributes for the benefit of creation. His goodness includes attributes such as **moral purity**, consisting of holiness, justice, and righteousness; **integrity**, flowing from His reality of speaking truth and proving true; **love**, bestowed in beauty, benevolence, grace, mercy, and persistence; and **stewardship**, exercising care aimed at fostering flourishing and fruitfulness in all creation.

God's intention was for humanity to walk in His likeness, demonstrating His goodness. People were created and intended to steward creation and tame the wild things as He would. The fall of humanity is most obvious is in the marring of God's likeness in us. Banished from walking with God in the cool of the garden and from observing how He modeled the conduct He desires, humanity does things God wouldn't do. We all fall short in acting like God in exercising moral purity, integrity, love and stewardship toward Him, one another, and all creation.

Fortunately, God returned at Jesus' incarnation, walked with humanity again, modeled desired behavior, and showed you how He would have you live in His likeness. The Holy Spirit then had the record of Jesus' teaching and conduct preserved for you to study. That's what we'll do in looking at Mark's Gospel.

Gender

With this background in mind, you can see that both genders have the potential to manifest God's image and likeness. Gender does not preclude thinking in accord with God's greatness and exercising God-like good behavior.

A Constant Call to Reflection

God has given the assignment to heal the body, teach the soul, and speak to the spirit of patients to Christians with a healthcare vocation. Christians in healthcare are not superior to any other Christians, but this particular calling means they certainly do have a privileged position! With privilege comes responsibility. Exercising that responsibility well requires introspection, meditation, and reflection.

As you go through this study of the Gospel of Mark, keep asking yourself these questions as they relate to your current and future practice of Christian healthcare:

1. Jesus quoted the proverb, "Doctor, heal yourself." (Luke 4:23). What is God telling you that you must have healed within yourself in preparation to serve God and people through your medical ministry?

2. As you read each account in the Gospel of Mark, what do you see God doing in the lives of all the people who appear, including patients, family members, bystanders, and the disciples? How can you incorporate what you observe into practicing medicine in His likeness?

3. John Stott taught that human history with God may be divided into four epochs: creation, the fall, redemption, and the consummation of all things. These four stages of God's relationship to humanity have implications for decision-making and the practice of Christian healthcare.

   - Creation: What was God's original intention for humans – body, soul, and spirit?

   - The Fall: What is bent or broken in your patient relative to God's intent? Look below the surface. Do they need to be taught something new to change how their soul thinks about, cares for, or uses their body? Is the patient actually dealing with a spiritual issue?

   - Redemption: What can be restored or brought closer to what God had in mind through the healing and/or teaching ministry? Put another way, what wild things are you able to tame as God's steward?

   - Consummation: What will God bring about in His final healing of those who accept Jesus by God's grace, through faith in the person and work of Jesus?

> How might your speaking of God's purposes, plans, and promises bring eternal hope and joy to what otherwise might be seen as a meaningless, hopeless, and joyless situation?

Medicine isn't always clear cut. Decisions aren't always easy to make. When faced with challenging situations, ask yourself how you may be guided to a godly decision by filtering the situation through the four stages of humanity's relationship to God.

A Word About Preaching and Speaking

In the HCSB texts used throughout the study, the translators accurately translated the Greek for talk about the things of God as "preach" or "preaching." In this study, to "speak to the spirit" carries the same connotation of proclaiming the things of God, while simultaneously emphasizing that your role is to *expose* Jesus to patients, rather than be perceived as *imposing* Jesus on patients.

A Final Comment -- Please Read the Text Afresh

Many of you have been believers for some time. You've read the Bible over and over. Accounts you'll read in Mark may seem old hat and familiar. Yet the actions and words of Jesus, to those who saw and heard them, were considered authoritative, amazing, and astonishing. They still are! If they seem mundane it may because you are reading superficially.

1. Read every word. The Holy Spirt used descriptive language to reveal physical and spiritual lessons that remain highly relevant to your healthcare practice.

2. Watch for signs. Mark's Gospel is rich in physical objects and actions intended to point to spiritual lessons. Body language and placement, clothes, settings, village names, etc. all have something to say and to teach you.

The Format Of This Book

Chapter Studies

The chapter divisions in Mark are interesting. Chapter breaks weren't inspired by the Holy Spirit. You don't find them in the early manuscripts and they weren't in the autograph. Chapter and verse divisions and markings were added later by others so that anyone would be able to cite Scripture that others could then find for themselves.

In the Gospel of Mark, generally speaking the chapter breaks fall in helpful locations. The stories recorded within the chapters fit together into a theme. It makes sense they form a chapter. That's the case in 14 of Mark's 16 chapters. However, I have chosen to break chapter one into two chapters of this book because the lessons taught by the two sides of the division are somewhat different. I've also chosen to break Mark 4-5 in a slightly different location for the same reason. Thus this book consists of 17 studies for 16 Gospel chapters.

Mapping the Path Forward

Each of the studies begins with a preamble called "Mapping the Path Forward." This is where major themes of the chapter are described and clues are given about important lessons to be found within the study.

In His Sandals

Each study consists of one module for each account, story, parable, etc. The module opens with the complete biblical text for reference, and then a series of comments or questions. Each module includes white space to write your answers, thoughts, or your own questions. It is possible to explore one module at a time for devotional study, select a few for a short group study, or complete all of the modules in order to grasp the larger themes of the study.

It is important to keep two ideas in mind when completing a module. First, context matters. While each module teaches a lesson and can stand alone, 'cherry-picking' modules means you will miss out on larger themes. The Holy Spirit and Mark put these texts in the order they are in, and provided the information they do, because they had an overarching purpose for the material in sum that you may not discover looking at only a few parts.

Second, effort matters. Certainly there are comments where they are appropriate, but this isn't a book designed to spoon feed the reader. It is a study crafted to draw you into the text, that you might then draw out of it new insights to the person and work of Jesus, particularly as it applies to the practice of healthcare. Hopefully you are not the sort of practitioner who speeds through or glosses over learning a new procedure or treatment. These studies are intended to change the way you view and care for your patients; study them as though you are learning a new technique.

Reflection

After the modules are all completed, take time to reflect upon what you've learned. This is the space to synthesize. Students doing these studies often find their big takeaways in this section.

Walking in Jesus' Footsteps Immediately

"Faith without deeds..." or "be doers, not just hearers" are familiar biblical principles. This section gives you one or more recommendations for something you can do not only to solidify your understanding of the material, but to apply it right away. The recommendations aren't the only things you can do to use the material. They are pump-primers. Let the Holy Spirit be your guide for lifetime use of what you learn, appropriate to your context and situation.

Supplemental Text References

Throughout these studies, you will encounter text references embedded in the questions or comments. Those which are printed in bold type (e.g., **Romans 10:3**) are very important to making the case or answering the question. You are strongly encouraged to read them. Those references in printed in plain type (e.g., Matthew 9:35-10:15) are relevant or illuminating, but not essential to read if you are short on time.

A Harmony of the Gospels

At the end of this book is the outline of *A Harmony of the Gospels* published in 1922 by professor A.T. Robertson. It is a very useful tool for seeing where a passage in Mark fits into Jesus' three-year ministry, or discovering what other Gospel writers had to say about events or sayings Mark recorded.

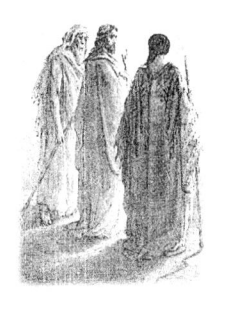

MARK 1:1-15

PREPARE THE WAY: THE MESSIAH IS HERE!

Mapping the Path Forward

Chapter one of the Gospel of Mark sets the stage for many of the themes and ideas that will appear throughout the Gospel and this book. In fact, so many important topics appear in this chapter, it is divided into two studies.

In this study of the first 15 verses of chapter one, there are several things to look out for. It is not enough to just notice them. Give serious thought to what God wants to teach you about being a follower of Jesus Christ. Ask yourself how what you are observing can be applied to uniquely practicing Christian healthcare.

Here are some of the many things to watch for in this study:

- Not only does God want to redeem people from their sins, but uncounted numbers of people want that redemption. As God's servant and herald, you have an important role in facilitating the introduction of sinners to the Savior.

- John the Baptist wore rugged camel hair and leather. His clothes are one of many examples where physical objects or actions are mentioned in Mark's Gospel that point to spiritual lessons, such as humility and an understanding of the role of a servant vis-à-vis Jesus the Master. The Apostle John called these signs. Watch for signs. The Holy Spirit uses them to teach. (Hint: In this study, look for a dove.)

- People come to you for help and hope. To the extent you can, you give it by healing and teaching. As a Christian healthcare practitioner, you should be eager to give eternal hope whenever the Holy Spirit leads you to. It is a profound privilege and a distinctive of your practice.

Jesus as Savior, John as Servant
(Mark 1:1-8)

1 ¹*The beginning of the gospel of Jesus Christ, the Son of God. ² As it is written in Isaiah the prophet:*

Look, I am sending My messenger ahead of You, who will prepare Your way.
³ A voice of one crying out in the wilderness: Prepare the way for the Lord; make His paths straight!

⁴ John came baptizing in the wilderness and preaching a baptism of repentance for the forgiveness of sins. ⁵ The whole Judean countryside and all the people of Jerusalem were flocking to him, and they were baptized by him in the Jordan River as they confessed their sins. ⁶ John wore a camel-hair garment with a leather belt around his waist and ate locusts and wild honey. ⁷ He was preaching: "Someone more powerful than I will come after me. I am not worthy to stoop down and untie the strap of His sandals. ⁸ I have baptized you with water, but He will baptize you with the Holy Spirit."

Mark uses prophesy, narrative, and quotations to describe and identify the Messiah who has come. What does this passage teach you about the person and work of Jesus?

How is Jesus' herald and servant, John the Baptist, described?

What attitudes for a servant of God does this model for you?

Which of these attitudes do you need help adopting?

The Holy Spirit and Healthcare
(Mark 1:8-13)

⁸ *I have baptized you with water, but He will baptize you with the Holy Spirit."*

⁹ *In those days Jesus came from Nazareth in Galilee and was baptized in the Jordan by John.* ¹⁰ *As soon as He came up out of the water, He saw the heavens being torn open and the Spirit descending to Him like a dove.* ¹¹ *And a voice came from heaven:*

"You are My beloved Son; I take delight in You!"

¹² *Immediately the Spirit drove Him into the wilderness.* ¹³ *He was in the wilderness 40 days, being tempted by Satan. He was with the wild animals, and the angels began to serve Him.*

You might wonder if Jesus was repenting of sin. As 1 John 3:5 states, Jesus had no sin. This baptismal act is pointing in part to Jesus taking your sins upon Himself and dying under wrath in your stead (Isaiah 53:11 and 1 Peter 2:24). **Matthew 3:13-15** says the only way people are able to fulfill all righteousness is to identify with Jesus' baptismal sign.

From Mark 1:8, 12, and **Matthew 3:16-17**, what additional event do you see accompanied Jesus' baptism? Immediately, what was the relationship between Jesus and the Holy Spirit?

What does this relational model between Jesus and the Holy Spirit suggest to you about the authority and importance the Holy Spirit should have in your life and healthcare ministry?

Rejoicing and Repenting
(Mark 1:14-15)

^{14} After John was arrested, Jesus went to Galilee, preaching the good news of God: ^{15} "The time is fulfilled, and the kingdom of God has come near. Repent and believe in the good news!"

How did Jesus frame His speaking the message of God – as a message of condemnation or good news? For a good example of how Jesus framed God's message, read **John 3:14-18**.

If you are walking in God's likeness as His disciples, how should you present the person and work of Jesus?

Jesus said the kingdom of God was near. Think about that. Kingdoms have kings on thrones reigning over loyal subjects. Is Jesus reigning on the throne of your heart? If not, why?

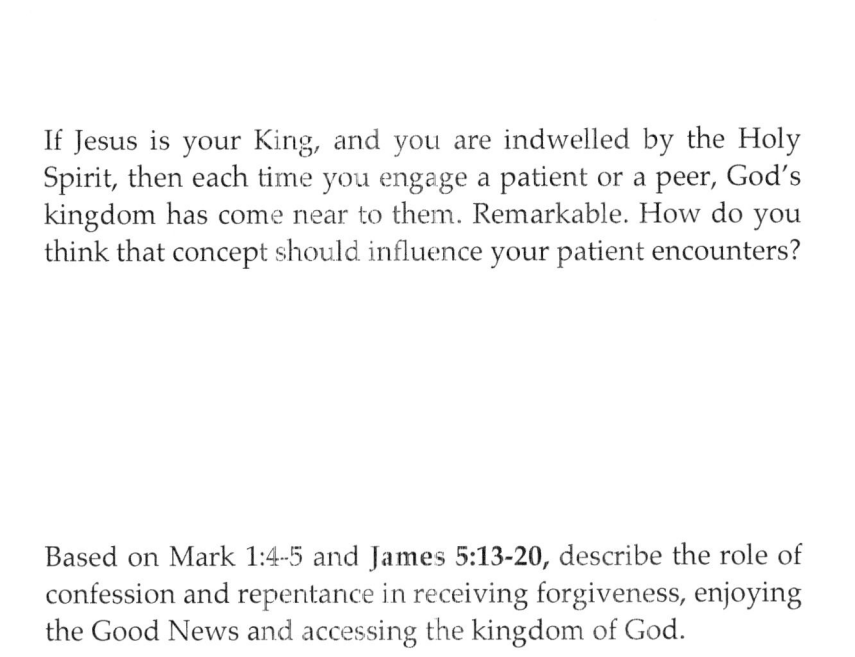

If Jesus is your King, and you are indwelled by the Holy Spirit, then each time you engage a patient or a peer, God's kingdom has come near to them. Remarkable. How do you think that concept should influence your patient encounters?

Based on Mark 1:4-5 and **James 5:13-20,** describe the role of confession and repentance in receiving forgiveness, enjoying the Good News and accessing the kingdom of God.

List at least two ways you can imagine confession and repentance being a part of your healthcare ministry

Reflection

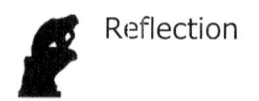

Which of these situations resonated the most with you? Explain why.

In what way does adopting God's perspective on Jesus and His servants change how you see yourself?

How do you envision this study of Mark 1:1-15 improving the way you will practice Christian healthcare?

Walking in Jesus' Footsteps Immediately

Jesus said His coming and calling on people to repent of their sins was good news. His servant, John the Baptist, proclaimed God's forgiveness for those who repent.

Write an outline of how you might explain to someone that while we all sin and fall short of the glory of God, God has good news. Jesus came to forgive us! Write the outline in a way that, as you say it, the opportunity for repentance sounds like good news.

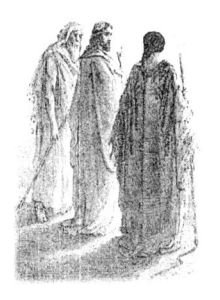

Mark 1:16-45

The Privileged Position Of Christians In Healthcare

Mapping the Path Forward

This study of the last 29 verses of Mark one consists of six modules. Each module has at least one foundational lesson to transform your Christian healthcare practice.

What does this study have to say to Christians in healthcare?

- The time of the prophets is past. The time of disciples – you – has come. Observe who calls and leads whom in a Master-disciple relationship.

- Authority has a double meaning: the right to direct, and the ability to enforce or empower. How will you engage with and exercise authority in your Christian practice?

- In a mysterious way, the Lord our God is one God of three persons. Reflecting His image somewhat, a human being consists of three parts: a body, soul, and spirit. Jesus immediately begins demonstrating to His disciples that He intends and has the ability to minister to each part, with excellence. Pay attention. He's going to give this assignment to you too.

- What's your purpose? Jesus knew His. He was very busy doing good things but He makes clear to His disciples that good things cannot be allowed to prevent them from fulfilling their God-given purpose.

Fishers of Men
(Mark 1:16-20)

¹⁶ As He was passing along by the Sea of Galilee, He saw Simon and Andrew, Simon's brother. They were casting a net into the sea, since they were fishermen.

¹⁷ "Follow Me," Jesus told them, "and I will make you fish for people!" ¹⁸ Immediately they left their nets and followed Him. ¹⁹ Going on a little farther, He saw James the son of Zebedee and his brother John. They were in their boat mending their nets. ²⁰ Immediately He called them, and they left their father Zebedee in the boat with the hired men and followed Him.

Who calls whom to become fishers of men?

Who empowers people to be fishers of men?

What is the single described prerequisite for becoming a fisher of men?

What does this prerequisite "Follow Me" mean to and for you? Give a thoughtful answer.

The Issue of Authority
(Mark 1:21-22)

²¹ Then they went into Capernaum, and right away He entered the synagogue on the Sabbath and began to teach. ²² They were astonished at His teaching because, unlike the scribes, He was teaching them as one having authority.

Jesus has just recruited His first disciples and begins training them. He is laying the foundation for how ministry in His name will be done for the entire age of the Gentiles. Mark records the first thing that needed to be established was the role and source of authority.

What was the first and continuously captivating characteristic of Jesus' ministry?

Through your role in healthcare, you already have a unique degree of authority in people's lives, too. Who else can order people to strip off their clothes, or 'bend over,' or 'turn your head and cough,' or 'open wide' and people just comply?

What will you do with this human authority – use it for the maximum good or squander it?

What would you do with God-given authority to speak on spiritual matters as a disciple of Christ Jesus?

Read **Matthew 28:16-20** and **Matthew 9:35-10:15**.

How much authority did and does Jesus have?

Does Jesus impute His authority to His disciples?

Looking at these passages carefully, what might the disciples have doubted?

What was Jesus' response to their doubts?

Teaching The Soul
(Mark 1:23-28)

²³ Just then a man with an unclean spirit was in their synagogue. He cried out, ²⁴ "What do You have to do with us, Jesus—Nazarene? Have You come to destroy us? I know who You are—the Holy One of God!"

²⁵ But Jesus rebuked him and said, "Be quiet, and come out of him!" ²⁶ And the unclean spirit convulsed him, shouted with a loud voice, and came out of him.

²⁷ Then they were all amazed, so they began to argue with one another, saying, "What is this? A new teaching with authority! He commands even the unclean spirits, and they obey Him." ²⁸ News about Him then spread throughout the entire vicinity of Galilee.

Review the meaning of 'soul' in Preliminary Points.

What are the four elements of which the soul consists?

- E_____
- I_____
- M_____
- W_____

What is the key responsibility of the soul?

Does Jesus care whether a person's soul is free of bondage? Explain why you gave the answer you did.

What link(s) do you see between setting the soul right and it exercising authority as God intended?

What effect did Jesus' teaching the soul of an individual and restoring its authority over the body have on the witnesses?

Healing the Body
(Mark 1:29-34)

²⁹ As soon as they left the synagogue, they went into Simon and Andrew's house with James and John. ³⁰ Simon's mother-in-law was lying in bed with a fever, and they told Him about her at once. ³¹ So He went to her, took her by the hand, and raised her up. The fever left her, and she began to serve them.

³² When evening came, after the sun had set, they began bringing to Him all those who were sick and those who were demon-possessed. ³³ The whole town was assembled at the door, ³⁴ and He healed many who were sick with various diseases and drove out many demons. But He would not permit the demons to speak, because they knew Him.

Review the meaning of 'body' in Preliminary Points.

Why are humans given a body, rather than being intangible ethereal beings?

Jesus was able to bring relief and, in some cases, miraculous cures of sickness and illness. What does it mean, however, that the healings were temporary – everyone healed would still someday die?

If everyone who gets healed will someday die anyway, is it futile or pointless to heal, or might healing still have value as a step toward a greater meaning and purpose? Explain.

Imagine being an oncologist who treats a patient pool where only 5% of her patients survive five years from time of diagnosis. How would your answer to the question above influence the way you felt about the value and importance of your practice? Would you want to quit or seek a greater purpose for your medical ministry?

Speaking to the Spirit – The Purpose Revealed (Mark 1:35-38)

³⁵ Very early in the morning, while it was still dark, He got up, went out, and made His way to a deserted place. And He was praying there. ³⁶ Simon and his companions went searching for Him. ³⁷ They found Him and said, "Everyone's looking for You!"

³⁸ And He said to them, "Let's go on to the neighboring villages so that I may preach there too. This is why I have come." ³⁹ So He went into all of Galilee, preaching in their synagogues and driving out demons.

Review the meaning of 'spirit' in Preliminary Points.

In your own words, describe the essential nature of the spirit that makes it distinct from the soul.

If Jesus' purpose was to make sick souls and broken bodies well, in the end, He failed. People He healed still died. Countless others were never healed. This is critical for you to grasp early in your healthcare ministry. For your ministry to be counted as truly successful, you must use the same benchmark for success that the Messiah Jesus used: fulfilling His true purpose. Countless practitioners fail to recognize this, subsequently becoming discouraged when their patients don't get better or they die.

From this passage, what was Jesus' purpose for coming to live among the people, teaching their souls and healing their bodies? Write out what you believe was His purpose statement.

Being Deliberate to Fulfill Your Purpose (Mark 1:40-45)

⁴⁰ Then a man with a serious skin disease came to Him and, on his knees, begged Him: "If You are willing, You can make me clean."

⁴¹ Moved with compassion, Jesus reached out His hand and touched him. "I am willing," He told him. "Be made clean." ⁴² Immediately the disease left him, and he was healed. ⁴³ Then He sternly warned him and sent him away at once, ⁴⁴ telling him, "See that you say nothing to anyone; but go and show yourself to the priest, and offer what Moses prescribed for your cleansing, as a testimony to them." ⁴⁵ Yet he went out and began to proclaim it widely and to spread the news, with the result that Jesus could no longer enter a town openly. But He was out in deserted places, and they would come to Him from everywhere.

Obviously Jesus was compassionate and willing to teach and heal. However, when the instruments to fulfill a purpose *become* the purpose, the true and primary purpose can get overwhelmed and pushed aside. That's a major reason you frequently see Jesus telling people and demons not to advertise His power to heal and teach.

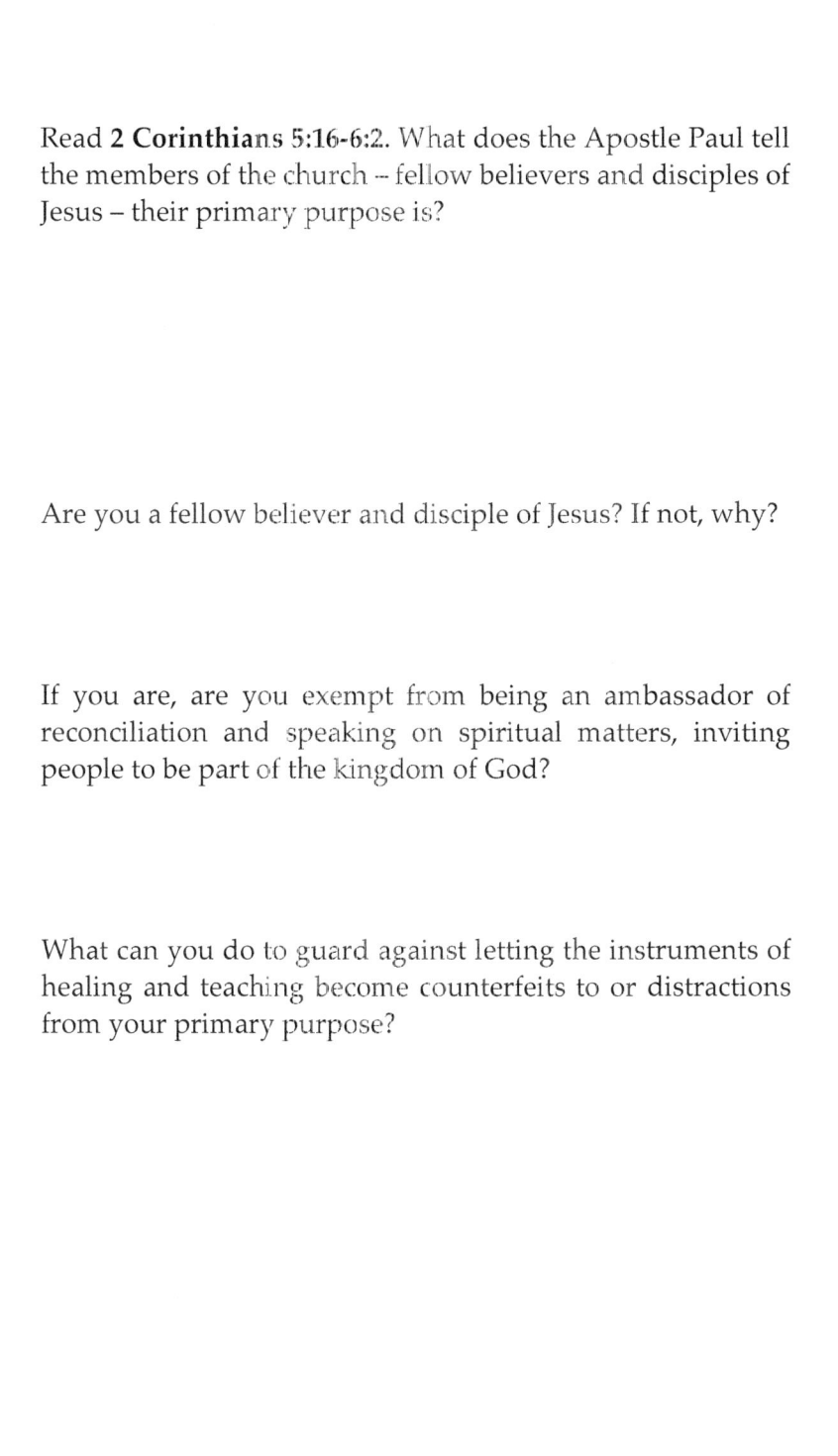

Read **2 Corinthians** 5:16-6:2. What does the Apostle Paul tell the members of the church -- fellow believers and disciples of Jesus – their primary purpose is?

Are you a fellow believer and disciple of Jesus? If not, why?

If you are, are you exempt from being an ambassador of reconciliation and speaking on spiritual matters, inviting people to be part of the kingdom of God?

What can you do to guard against letting the instruments of healing and teaching become counterfeits to or distractions from your primary purpose?

Reflection

Christians in healthcare are not superior to any other Christians. However, they are in a uniquely privileged position because through Christian healthcare they can walk in Jesus' footsteps. In one encounter, through Christian healthcare, they are able to _____ the soul, _____ the body, and _____ to the spirit.

Serving Jesus, you are closest to following in His footsteps when you make His _____ yours, too.

Serving others through healthcare, you serve Jesus under His _____, given to you as His follower.

Walking in His footsteps, empowered by His _____, and focused by His Word, He will make you a _____ ____ _____.

Walking in Jesus' Footsteps Immediately

In light of what you've learned in this study, write out your own purpose statement as a Christian healthcare practitioner. Make it an offering to God.

Mark 2

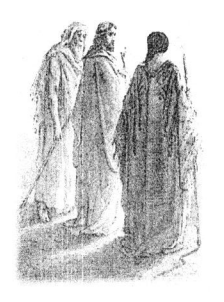

Exploding The Expected Order Of Things

Mapping the Path Forward

A cursory glance at this chapter suggests a series of events without any real theme. But in reality, the chapter is unified by one overarching observation: Jesus came to explode the rigid legalism and narrow view of spiritual life held by religious people.

This study has plenty to say to Christians in healthcare.

- Keep an eye out for Jesus' priorities – if you are following in His footsteps, they should become your priorities, too.

- Check your own heart for how you view (judge) people who are not like you. Does Jesus see them as you might be seeing them?

- What does this chapter say about how Jesus values caring for the whole person – body, soul and spirit? How will this impact your view of patient care?

- Who are Jesus' audiences in these encounters? Consider how often your patients are not the only ones hanging on your words.

The Son of Man Forgives and Heals
(Mark 2:1-12)

2 ¹*When He entered Capernaum again after some days, it was reported that He was at home. ² So many people gathered together that there was no more room, not even in the doorway, and He was speaking the message to them. ³ Then they came to Him bringing a paralytic, carried by four men. ⁴ Since they were not able to bring him to Jesus because of the crowd, they removed the roof above where He was. And when they had broken through, they lowered the mat on which the paralytic was lying.*

⁵ *Seeing their faith, Jesus told the paralytic, "Son, your sins are forgiven."*

⁶ *But some of the scribes were sitting there, thinking to themselves:* ⁷ *"Why does He speak like this? He's blaspheming! Who can forgive sins but God alone?"*

⁸ *Right away Jesus understood in His spirit that they were thinking like this within themselves and said to them, "Why are you thinking these things in your hearts?* ⁹ *Which is easier: to say to the paralytic, 'Your sins are forgiven,' or to say, 'Get up, pick up your mat, and walk'?* ¹⁰ *But so you may know that the Son of Man has authority on earth to forgive sins," He told the paralytic,* ¹¹ *"I tell you: get up, pick up your mat, and go home."*

¹² *Immediately he got up, picked up the mat, and went out in front of everyone. As a result, they were all astounded and gave glory to God, saying, "We have never seen anything like this!"*

What was Jesus' priority, even as crowds filled the house?

Why do you think friends brought the paralytic to Jesus?

Mark records in verse 4 the highly disruptive and somewhat destructive act of ripping the roof off to get to Jesus. Read **Matthew 11:12**. What thoughts or questions do you have after reading these two passages side-by-side?

What was the first thing Jesus did for the paralytic?

What do you think was motivating Jesus to act in the way and order that He did?

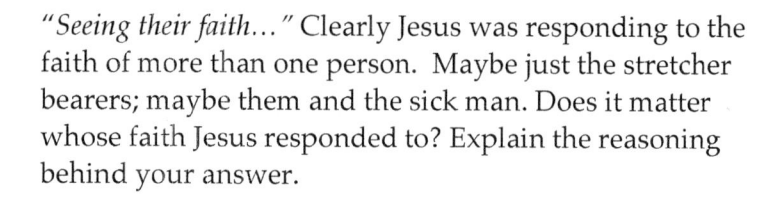

"Seeing their faith..." Clearly Jesus was responding to the faith of more than one person. Maybe just the stretcher bearers; maybe them and the sick man. Does it matter whose faith Jesus responded to? Explain the reasoning behind your answer.

How do you see faith fitting into your patient care?

Though Jesus' ultimate priority was forgiving sins of those who had faith, notice that He bolstered the authority of His message to the audience by healing the body of the paralytic. What does this say to you about the importance of your studies, continuing education, and excellent patient care?

The Son of Man Calls Sick Sinners
(Mark 2:13-17)

[13] *Then Jesus went out again beside the sea. The whole crowd was coming to Him, and He taught them.* [14] *Then, moving on, He saw Levi the son of Alphaeus sitting at the tax office, and He said to him, "Follow Me!" So he got up and followed Him.*

[15] *While He was reclining at the table in Levi's house, many tax collectors and sinners were also guests with Jesus and His disciples, because there were many who were following Him.* [16] *When the scribes of the Pharisees saw that He was eating with sinners and tax collectors, they asked His disciples, "Why does He eat with tax collectors and sinners?"*

[17] *When Jesus heard this, He told them, "Those who are well don't need a doctor, but the sick do need one. I didn't come to call the righteous, but sinners."*

In the first twelve verses of Mark 2, Jesus healed bodies and spoke to spirits. In verse 13, He completed His triplex method of care by teaching _____.

Matthew was counted among a despised gathering of tax collectors and sinners. What do verse 15 and **2 Peter 3:9** say about why Jesus was found dining with them?

If your healthcare ministry is modeled after Jesus, what does this say about how you should relate to 'undesirables' who enter your practice seeking care?

Comment on what verse 17 says to you.

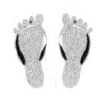

You Don't Have to Destroy Everything to Have Something New
(Mark 2:18-22)

¹⁸ Now John's disciples and the Pharisees were fasting. People came and asked Him, "Why do John's disciples and the Pharisees' disciples fast, but Your disciples do not fast?"

¹⁹ Jesus said to them, "The wedding guests cannot fast while the groom is with them, can they? As long as they have the groom with them, they cannot fast. ²⁰ But the time will come when the groom is taken away from them, and then they will fast in that day. ²¹ No one sews a patch of unshrunk cloth on an old garment. Otherwise, the new patch pulls away from the old cloth, and a worse tear is made. ²² And no one puts new wine into old wineskins. Otherwise, the wine will burst the skins, and the wine is lost as well as the skins. But new wine is for fresh wineskins."

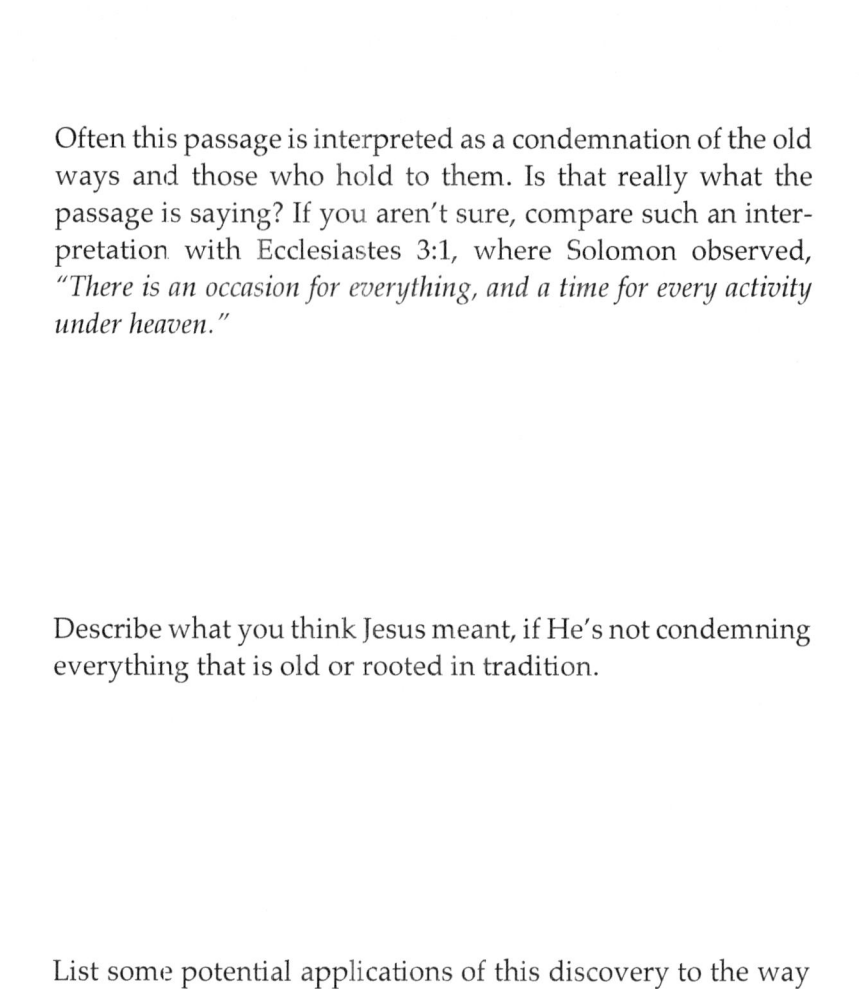

Often this passage is interpreted as a condemnation of the old ways and those who hold to them. Is that really what the passage is saying? If you aren't sure, compare such an interpretation with Ecclesiastes 3:1, where Solomon observed, *"There is an occasion for everything, and a time for every activity under heaven."*

Describe what you think Jesus meant, if He's not condemning everything that is old or rooted in tradition.

List some potential applications of this discovery to the way you might practice patient care.

Having God's Perspective
(Mark 2:23-28)

²³ On the Sabbath He was going through the grainfields, and His disciples began to make their way picking some heads of grain. ²⁴ The Pharisees said to Him, "Look, why are they doing what is not lawful on the Sabbath?"

²⁵ He said to them, "Have you never read what David and those who were with him did when he was in need and hungry— ²⁶ how he entered the house of God in the time of Abiathar the high priest and ate the sacred bread—which is not lawful for anyone to eat except the priests—and also gave some to his companions?" ²⁷ Then He told them, "The Sabbath was made for man and not man for the Sabbath. ²⁸ Therefore, the Son of Man is Lord even of the Sabbath."

In healthcare, there is certainly a need for best practices, standards of care, protocols, policies and procedures, and the like. Occasionally, however, you will encounter a patient who didn't read them. You may be confronted with a choice between following the rules no matter what and stepping out of your comfort zone in order to act in the patient's best interest.

How do you envision handling such challenging situations?

Reflection

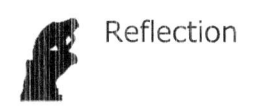

Which of the four vignettes resonated most with you? Explain why.

How will this study alter the way you will provide Christian healthcare to your patients?

Did this study expose any ungodly thinking or prejudices you might have? If so, name them. What will you do to change your thinking to be godly?

Walking in Jesus' Footsteps Immediately

Think carefully about all the different audiences you have during your week, whether at school, work, church, home, or other social gatherings. Are there any that the Holy Spirit is telling you that you have neglected or shunned?

Make and carry out a plan to reach out with the love of Jesus to those you've neglected or shunned. In doing so, make sure they hear from you something about the love of Jesus. Just being nice to them isn't enough to say you reached out to them as Jesus would.

One might argue that if you're not willing to reach out to a shunned or neglected neighbor with the love of Jesus, you are not really ready to take God's love around the globe.

Mark 3

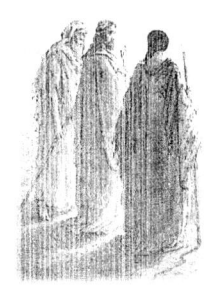

The Irony Of Opposition To Healing Ministry

Mapping the Path Forward

The honeymoon is over. In this chapter Mark records that everywhere Jesus turned He encountered opposition. Yet, sure of His mission, Jesus persevered in the face of every opponent.

What does this study have to say to Christians in healthcare?

- The right of conscience for healthcare workers is under fire today. How did Jesus respond to the people and structures which opposed Him, acting in accord with what He believed was right?

- Being excellent at healing can make you *too* popular. It creates some unique risks. Notice how Jesus prepared for an enduring ministry.

- Not everyone on your teams with whom you work are your allies. You need to think about how Jesus dealt with a potential traitor on His team.

- How is your own spiritual health? Are you working against yourself and the best interests of your patients by not tending to it?

- Who is your family – your support network in the face of opposition?

Making Decisions of Conscience
(Mark 3:1-6)

3 ¹*Now He entered the synagogue again, and a man was there who had a paralyzed hand.* ²*In order to accuse Him, they were watching Him closely to see whether He would heal him on the Sabbath.* ³*He told the man with the paralyzed hand, "Stand before us."* ⁴*Then He said to them, "Is it lawful on the Sabbath to do what is good or to do what is evil, to save life or to kill?" But they were silent.* ⁵*After looking around at them with anger and sorrow at the hardness of their hearts, He told the man, "Stretch out your hand." So he stretched it out, and his hand was restored.* ⁶*Immediately the Pharisees went out and started plotting with the Herodians against Him, how they might destroy Him.*

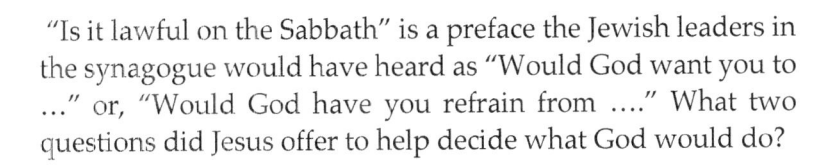

"Is it lawful on the Sabbath" is a preface the Jewish leaders in the synagogue would have heard as "Would God want you to …" or, "Would God have you refrain from …." What two questions did Jesus offer to help decide what God would do?

How might these two questions help you decide what is the correct action to take when faced with a moral dilemma or opposition to your Christian healthcare ministry?

What risk did Jesus take in making His decision to heal in the face of opposition?

Because Jesus knew what was the right thing to do, He did it despite risks. The night before Jesus was crucified, His disciple Peter thought he could do the same thing. He failed miserably. Yet Peter went on to become a pillar of the church. What event transformed Peter into a rock? (Hint: Acts 2)

Planning Not to Get Overrun and Burned Out (Mark 3:7-12)

⁷ Jesus departed with His disciples to the sea, and a large crowd followed from Galilee, Judea, ⁸ Jerusalem, Idumea, beyond the Jordan, and around Tyre and Sidon. The large crowd came to Him because they heard about everything He was doing. ⁹ Then He told His disciples to have a small boat ready for Him, so the crowd would not crush Him. ¹⁰ Since He had healed many, all who had diseases were pressing toward Him to touch Him. ¹¹ Whenever the unclean spirits saw Him, those possessed fell down before Him and cried out, "You are the Son of God!" ¹² And He would strongly warn them not to make Him known.

Describe what problems being an effective healer and teacher created for Jesus.

What provisions did Jesus make to protect His physical well-being and ongoing ministry? Give some real thought to this question before you answer it.

What steps might you take to protect your own well-being and ministry?

Passing on the Work···Who Do You Disciple? (Mark 3:13-19)

¹³ Then He went up the mountain and summoned those He wanted, and they came to Him. ¹⁴ He also appointed 12 — He also named them apostles — to be with Him, to send them out to preach, ¹⁵ and to have authority to drive out demons.

¹⁶ He appointed the Twelve:

To Simon, He gave the name Peter;
¹⁷ and to James the son of Zebedee,
and to his brother John,
He gave the name "Boanerges" (that is, "Sons of Thunder");
¹⁸ Andrew;
Philip and Bartholomew;
Matthew and Thomas;
James the son of Alphaeus, and Thaddaeus;
Simon the Zealot,
¹⁹ and Judas Iscariot,
who also betrayed Him.

In some manuscripts, verse 15 reads, *"and to have authority to heal diseases and to drive out demons."* By way of review, that means Jesus sent the apostles out to: _____ the body, _____ the soul, and _____ to the spirit of people.

Did knowing that among His inner circle one would betray Him keep Jesus from discipling all twelve that He appointed to be apostles?

Contrast **Matthew 13:24-30** with **Acts 20:29-31**. According to these examples, when do you let someone who is not supportive of you or your team stay, and when must you banish them?

The Matter of Your Own Spiritual Health
(Mark 3:20-30)

²⁰ *Then He went home, and the crowd gathered again so that they were not even able to eat.* ²¹ *When His family heard this, they set out to restrain Him, because they said, "He's out of His mind."*

²² *The scribes who had come down from Jerusalem said, "He has Beelzebul in Him!" and, "He drives out demons by the ruler of the demons!"*

²³ *So He summoned them and spoke to them in parables: "How can Satan drive out Satan?* ²⁴ *If a kingdom is divided against itself, that kingdom cannot stand.* ²⁵ *If a house is divided against itself, that house cannot stand.* ²⁶ *And if Satan rebels against himself and is divided, he cannot stand but is finished!*

²⁷ *"On the other hand, no one can enter a strong man's house and rob his possessions unless he first ties up the strong man. Then he will rob his house.* ²⁸ *I assure you: People will be forgiven for all sins and whatever blasphemies they may blaspheme.* ²⁹ *But whoever blasphemes against the Holy Spirit never has forgiveness, but is guilty of an eternal sin"* — ³⁰ *because they were saying, "He has an unclean spirit."*

Not everyone will understand your motivations or actions. The important question is, do you do your own spiritual self-examinations, honestly testing your own understanding of your motivations and the actions which follow? Hopefully you do, for as the Apostle Paul says in 1 Corinthians 11, you should judge yourself, lest you be judged by God.

When you face opposition, are you motivated by your flesh and satanic temptations, or are you walking in God's Spirit and wisdom, when you respond? It will make a difference in whether your ministry honors God and redeems people.

If you've realized some of your responses to opposition have been ungodly, what will you do to make amends and prevent future similar responses?

Your Support Network in Tough Times (Mark 3:31-35)

³¹ Then His mother and His brothers came, and standing outside, they sent word to Him and called Him. ³² A crowd was sitting around Him and told Him, "Look, Your mother, Your brothers, and Your sisters are outside asking for You."

³³ He replied to them, "Who are My mother and My brothers?" ³⁴ And looking about at those who were sitting in a circle around Him, He said, "Here are My mother and My brothers! ³⁵ Whoever does the will of God is My brother and sister and mother."

As you have seen throughout this chapter, Jesus faced opposition for doing what was right – doing good and saving lives. All along the way though, He had a support team around Him. You will need one too. Begin cultivating relationships with fellow Christians in healthcare now. Don't let a hectic schedule or your own success cause you to abandon those relationships. Those people need you and you need them.

How many people can you list in healthcare that you would consider part of a support network when you face opposition or temptation?

Reflection

Which of these five modules resonated the most with you? Why?

Describe at least one incident where you responded to opposition from a peer or teammate in an ungodly way.

If you had it to do over again, how might you change your response to that same opposition?

Walking in Jesus' Footsteps Immediately

If you are in practice already, or considering a practice specialty, what are some of the moral or ethical pitfalls your specialty engenders? For example, if you are a geriatric or cardiology specialist, people might ask you to help them die. A urologist might be asked to participate in gender reassignment.

Choose one pitfall and write out how you envision responding in a godly way to opposition to your exercising your right of conscience and refusing to participate in something with which you disagree.

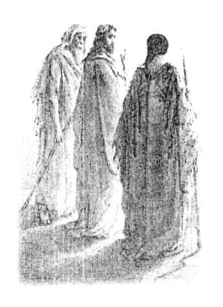

Mark 4:1-34

Parables Of What Are – And Aren't – Your Tasks

Mapping the Path Forward

Beginning in this chapter, Mark lays out some specific lessons Jesus began to teach His disciples. In your study here, He will use parables. God recorded and preserved these parables for your edification. Pray that the Holy Spirit will give you the illumination you need so that your eyes will see and your ears will hear, that you might have understanding.

Because this study is targeting Christians in healthcare in particular, the order of some of the passages has been changed to enhance the flow of the lessons related to them. No verses are left out or altered.

What does this study have to say to Christians in healthcare?

- There are certain responsibilities given to you to fulfill.

- There are also responsibilities that are not yours; some things belong to your patient and others belong to God.

- Your goal through this study should be to discern the difference and then commit to do what you have been tasked to do.

Parables, Prophets, and Disciples
(Mark 4:10-12, 33-34)

4 *¹⁰ When He was alone with the Twelve, those who were around Him asked Him about the parables. ¹¹ He answered them, "The secret of the kingdom of God has been given to you, but to those outside, everything comes in parables ¹² so that they may look and look,*
yet not perceive;
they may listen and listen,
yet not understand;
otherwise, they might turn back —
and be forgiven."

³³ He would speak the word to them with many parables like these, as they were able to understand. ³⁴ And He did not speak to them without a parable. Privately, however, He would explain everything to His own disciples.

After reading Mark 4:10-12 and **Matthew 13:10-15,** have you discovered that Jesus doesn't use parables as a joke or way to hide heaven? He uses them to reveal to Himself, bystanders, and to the person to whom He is speaking their heart condition and their willingness to accept His call to repentance and eternal life through the Gospel.

When Jesus spoke in parables, He got one of three responses, just as you will when you speak on spiritual matters. One response may be to reject or ignore your words. Another will be to understand and accept them. The third is to not fully understand but be curious. Presuming you appropriately speak spiritually in love, with gentleness and respect, you are not responsible for how people respond.

Should you feel guilty if your words aren't received with joy?

Read Mark 4:33-34 and **Matthew 13:16-17**.

Did God reveal to the prophets everything He was doing?

In teaching the disciples, was Jesus building upon what He told the prophets?

Should you expect God has told or will tell you everything He has done or is doing?

What is your responsibility regarding what you do know and understand?

The Parable of the Soils
(Mark 4:1-9, 13-20)

4 [1] *Again He began to teach by the sea, and a very large crowd gathered around Him. So He got into a boat on the sea and sat down, while the whole crowd was on the shore facing the sea.* [2] *He taught them many things in parables, and in His teaching He said to them:* [3] *"Listen! Consider the sower who went out to sow.* [4] *As he sowed, this occurred: Some seed fell along the path, and the birds came and ate it up.* [5] *Other seed fell on rocky ground where it didn't have much soil, and it sprang up right away, since it didn't have deep soil.* [6] *When the sun came up, it was scorched, and since it didn't have a root, it withered.* [7] *Other seed fell among thorns, and the thorns came up and choked it, and it didn't produce a crop.* [8] *Still others fell on good ground and produced a crop that increased 30, 60, and 100 times what was sown."* [9] *Then He said, "Anyone who has ears to hear should listen!"*

-----

[13] *Then He said to them: "Don't you understand this parable? How then will you understand any of the parables?* [14] *The sower sows the word.* [15] *These are the ones along the path where the word is sown: when they hear, immediately Satan comes and takes away the word sown in them.* [16] *And these are the ones sown on rocky ground: when they hear the word, immediately they receive it with joy.* [17] *But they have no root in themselves; they are short-lived. When pressure or persecution comes because of the word, they immediately stumble.* [18] *Others are sown among thorns; these are the ones who hear the word,* [19] *but the worries of this age, the seduction of wealth, and the desires for other things enter in and choke the word, and it becomes unfruitful.* [20] *But the ones sown on good ground are those who hear the word, welcome it, and produce a crop: 30, 60, and 100 times what was sown."*

What was the assigned task of the sower?

Jesus makes it very clear. What is the seed to be sown?

Describe each of the four soils and how you might recognize a person each soil-type represents.

Several years of working with and counseling Christians in healthcare suggests the greatest risk to them is becoming like the third type of soil. They can be so consumed by the things of this world they become unfruitful, at least so far as using their vocation of healthcare as ambassadors of reconciliation. What cares threaten to choke out your fruitfulness?

The Size of the Seed
(Mark 4:30-32)

30 And He said: "How can we illustrate the kingdom of God, or what parable can we use to describe it? 31 It's like a mustard seed that, when sown in the soil, is smaller than all the seeds on the ground. 32 And when sown, it comes up and grows taller than all the vegetables, and produces large branches, so that the birds of the sky can nest in its shade."

Do you have to sow big seeds to make a big difference?

If you are looking to reap a large harvest, which do you think is more important – the size of the seed or the number of seeds you sow?

Your Responsibility – and Not Your Responsibility
(Mark 4:26-29)

[26] "The kingdom of God is like this," He said. "A man scatters seed on the ground; [27] he sleeps and rises—night and day, and the seed sprouts and grows—he doesn't know how. [28] The soil produces a crop by itself—first the blade, then the head, and then the ripe grain on the head. [29] But as soon as the crop is ready, he sends for the sickle, because the harvest has come."

Name the one thing that this parable teaches IS NOT your responsibility.

List the two things that this parable teaches ARE your responsibility.

The parable teaches that occasionally a sower will recognize that a field is white unto harvest. Is the sower to ignore what they see? No! They are to call for the reaper.

Who is ultimately responsible for reaping the spiritual harvest? God, of course. Consider this though: as a believer, you are indwelled by the Holy Spirit. As a sower calling for the reaper, the reaper is in you and wants to use you.

Therefore, you must be ready to not only recognize the condition of the field, but listen to God as He empowers you and gives you the words to speak unto the one He is reaping.

When Does a Sower Sow?
(Mark 4:21-23)

21 He also said to them, "Is a lamp brought in to be put under a basket or under a bed? Isn't it to be put on a lampstand? 22 For nothing is concealed except to be revealed, and nothing hidden except to come to light. 23 If anyone has ears to hear, he should listen!"

Do farmers only work during daylight hours, when all looks sunny, or do they work in the dark too, before sunup and after sundown?

If it is the latter case, what does that teach you about being a light even if it appears you are going to be shining into darkness?

The Rule of Seeds
(Mark 4:24-25)

> ^{24} *Then He said to them, "Pay attention to what you hear. By the measure you use, it will be measured and added to you.* ^{25} *For to the one who has, it will be given, and from the one who does not have, even what he has will be taken away."*

To grasp the imperative that it is your job to sow, and that not sowing according to the Master's plan has consequences, please read the following passages and answer the questions.

Read **2 Corinthians 9:6-15**.

What is the attitude God desires from seed sowers?

Seed sowing for God is a partnership with God. List the benefits of partnering to sow seeds for God.

Read **Exodus 16**.

What seed is manna compared to?

List the benefits of gathering the manna according to God's schedule and plan.

Describe the consequence of harvesting manna and holding onto it rather than eating it. Compare this to what Jesus warned in Mark 4:25.

Read **Matthew 25:14-30**.

God will provide His servants seed. He's apparently not interested in how much seed He gives to different individuals, nor in how big their individual harvests are. However, God is keenly interested in and judges what?

The Rule of Seeds
The seed you sow is the crop that will grow;
The more you sow, the more that will grow;
The more you grow, the fuller your storehouse;
Food for now and continued bounty for the future.

Reflection

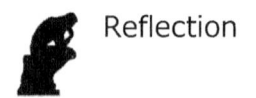

Describe the things in this study that got your attention. What made them important lessons for you?

Almost certainly this study raised some concerns about practicing healthcare and 'evangelizing.' Write out your concerns in the form of questions. After you complete the next two studies, review your questions and see if they have been answered.

Walking in Jesus' Footsteps Immediately

¹⁸ Others are sown among thorns; these are the ones who hear the word, ¹⁹ but the worries of this age, the seduction of wealth, and the desires for other things enter in and choke the word, and it becomes unfruitful.

You've been sown with the seed of God's Word. That is how you became a believer. The question is whether you are letting those things which compete for your time, treasure, and talents choke the fruitfulness for God right out of you?

What worry, seduction, or desire is the greatest hindrance or distraction keeping you from being more fruitful for God?

If you are willing, what concrete step(s) will you take to break that thing's chokehold on you?

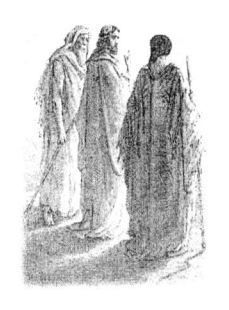

Mark 4:35-5:43

Tell Of Your Encounter With The Omnipotent One (Part 1)

Mapping the Path Forward

At the beginning of Mark 4, Jesus told parables as a way to reveal those who had calloused hearts and wouldn't hear His message. Now Jesus will use His surroundings as a canvas to reveal His omnipotence and demonstrate that the Lord's love and power is available to those who have faith in Him.

What will this study have to say to Christians in healthcare?

- These lessons do not preclude you doing your best to address your issues with the resources you have, even though they may be insufficient.

- There is nothing in creation over which Jesus doesn't have power. And nothing which He is unwilling to overcome to rescue people, especially once they've come to the end of themselves.

- The prescription for accessing His salvation, in all realms, is faith.

- Faith is God's gift (Ephesians 2:8-9); where that faith resides may vary.

Power Over All Physical Creation – Things Seen
(Mark 4:35-41)

^{35} On that day, when evening had come, He told them, "Let's cross over to the other side of the sea." ^{36} So they left the crowd and took Him along since He was already in the boat. And other boats were with Him. ^{37} A fierce windstorm arose, and the waves were breaking over the boat, so that the boat was already being swamped. ^{38} But He was in the stern, sleeping on the cushion. So they woke Him up and said to Him, "Teacher! Don't You care that we're going to die?"

^{39} He got up, rebuked the wind, and said to the sea, "Silence! Be still!" The wind ceased, and there was a great calm. ^{40} Then He said to them, "Why are you fearful? Do you still have no faith?"

^{41} And they were terrified and asked one another, "Who then is this? Even the wind and the sea obey Him!"

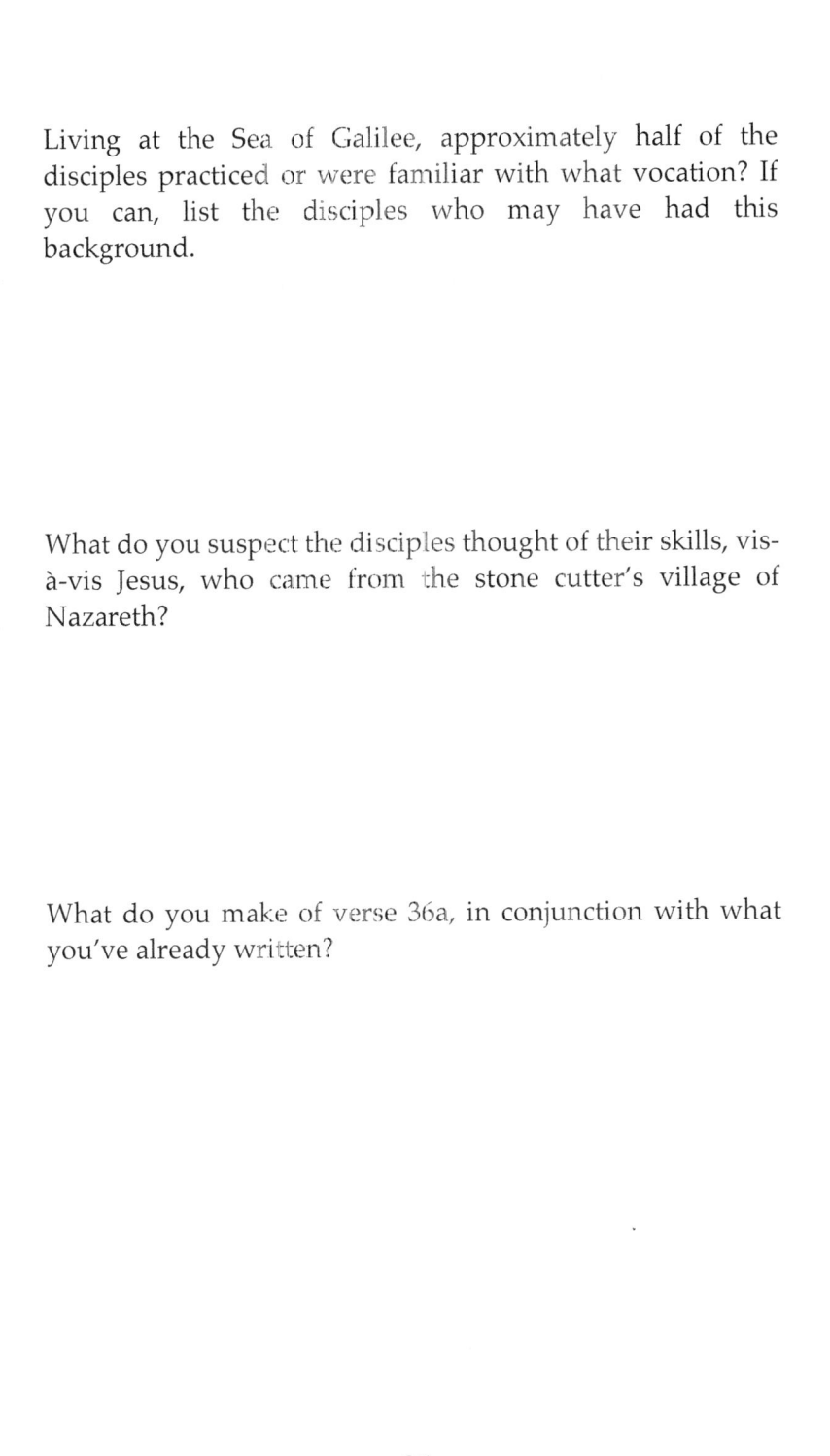

Living at the Sea of Galilee, approximately half of the disciples practiced or were familiar with what vocation? If you can, list the disciples who may have had this background.

What do you suspect the disciples thought of their skills, vis-à-vis Jesus, who came from the stone cutter's village of Nazareth?

What do you make of verse 36a, in conjunction with what you've already written?

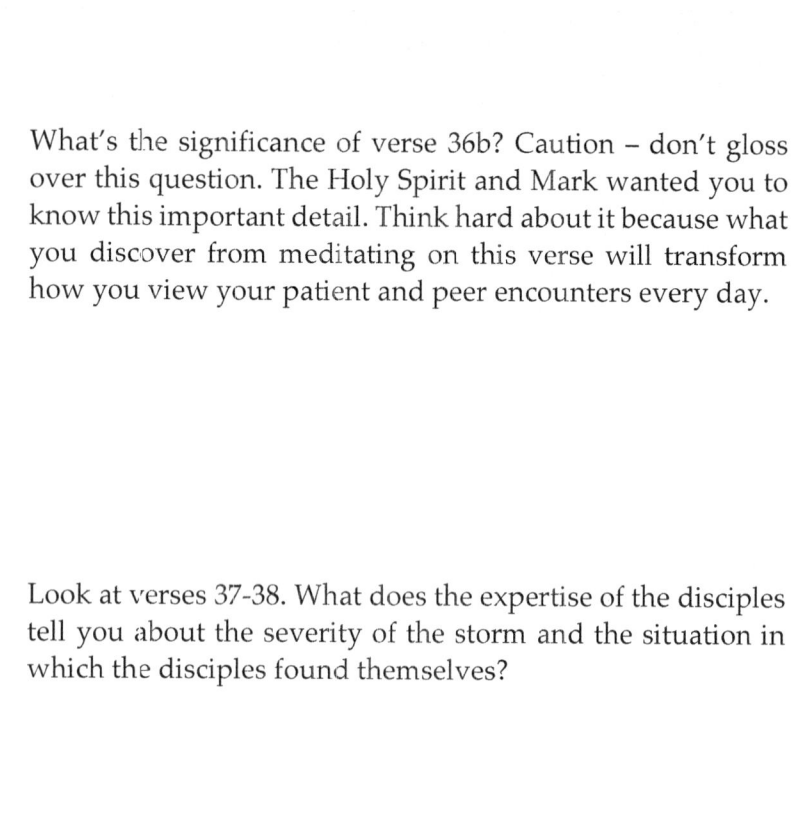

What's the significance of verse 36b? Caution – don't gloss over this question. The Holy Spirit and Mark wanted you to know this important detail. Think hard about it because what you discover from meditating on this verse will transform how you view your patient and peer encounters every day.

Look at verses 37-38. What does the expertise of the disciples tell you about the severity of the storm and the situation in which the disciples found themselves?

From a boating perspective, what might it mean that Jesus was resting at the stern?

From verse 40, what do you think the disciples were fearful of? Is this the same fear many patients express?

What should the disciples have been fearful of?

In what or whom does Jesus want them to have faith?

Many of the disciples were well-versed in Scripture (as you learn from reading the writings of Matthew, John, and Peter), suggesting they should have been at least familiar with **Psalm 65:5-8, 89:8-9, 107:23-32,** and **Isaiah 43:1-7**. Please take time now to read these four passages.

After you've read the four passages, how would you explain the disciples crying out in bewilderment about who Jesus is – even as they acknowledge Jesus just did what these Scripture passages attribute to God alone?

What does this account say to you about the importance of knowing and recalling God's Word in order to recognize Jesus' presence and who He actually is?

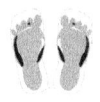

Power Over All Immaterial Creation – Things Unseen
(Mark 5:1-20)

5 *¹Then they came to the other side of the sea, to the region of the Gerasenes. ² As soon as He got out of the boat, a man with an unclean spirit came out of the tombs and met Him. ³ He lived in the tombs.* [Luke 8:27 adds the detail, *"For a long time he had worn no clothes...."*] *No one was able to restrain him anymore—even with chains—* ⁴ *because he often had been bound with shackles and chains, but had snapped off the chains and smashed the shackles. No one was strong enough to subdue him.* ⁵ *And always, night and day, he was crying out among the tombs and in the mountains and cutting himself with stones.*

⁶ *When he saw Jesus from a distance, he ran and knelt down before Him.* ⁷ *And he cried out with a loud voice, "What do You have to do with me, Jesus, Son of the Most High God? I beg You before God, don't torment me!"* ⁸ *For He had told him, "Come out of the man, you unclean spirit!"*

⁹ *"What is your name?" He asked him.*

"My name is Legion," he answered Him, "because we are many." ¹⁰ *And he kept begging Him not to send them out of the region.*

¹¹ *Now a large herd of pigs was there, feeding on the hillside.* ¹² *The demons begged Him, "Send us to the pigs, so we may enter them."* ¹³ *And He gave them permission. Then the unclean spirits came out and entered the pigs, and the herd of about 2,000 rushed down the steep bank into the sea and drowned there.* ¹⁴ *The men who tended then ran off and reported it in the town and the countryside, and people went to see what had happened.* ¹⁵ *They came to Jesus and saw the man who had been demon-possessed by the legion, sitting there, dressed and in his right mind; and they were afraid.*

¹⁶ The eyewitnesses described to them what had happened to the demon-possessed man and told about the pigs. ¹⁷ Then they began to beg Him to leave their region.

¹⁸ As He was getting into the boat, the man who had been demon-possessed kept begging Him to be with Him. ¹⁹ But He would not let him; instead, He told him, "Go back home to your own people, and report to them how much the Lord has done for you and how He has had mercy on you." ²⁰ So he went out and began to proclaim in the Decapolis how much Jesus had done for him, and they were all amazed.

The first eight verses of this passage suggest this man's entire humanity was in grave trouble: body, soul, and spirit. Break down what his issues were:

Body:

Soul:

Spirit:

Recall that the soul is what makes every human utterly unique, consisting of the e_____, i_____, m_____, and w_____. All of the behavioral indicators point to this man being sick in his soul. But Jesus uses His Divine discernment to recognize in this man's case, his real rescue required a supernatural spiritual intervention.

As a Christian in healthcare, caring for people as Jesus did – body, soul and spirit – what does this mean for your personal preparation and training to practice Christian healthcare?

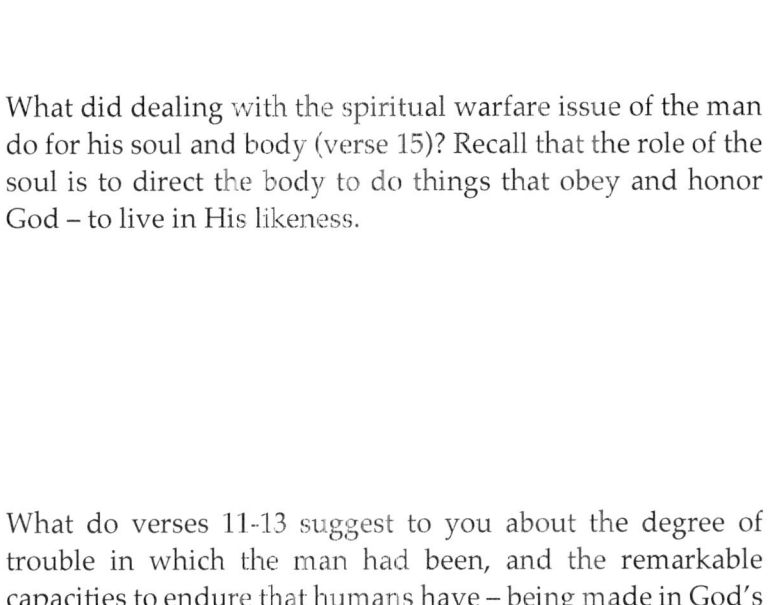

What did dealing with the spiritual warfare issue of the man do for his soul and body (verse 15)? Recall that the role of the soul is to direct the body to do things that obey and honor God – to live in His likeness.

What do verses 11-13 suggest to you about the degree of trouble in which the man had been, and the remarkable capacities to endure that humans have – being made in God's image and likeness – compared to animals?

Did everyone around the situation understand what Jesus was doing? What was their seemingly universal response to Jesus' ministry?

CRITICAL QUESTIONS

What two specific things did Jesus direct this healed man to tell those people who knew him?

    1.

    2.

Was the healed man told by Jesus that he had to: mention sin, death, repentance, blood, Hell or Heaven, or the plan of salvation; hand out tracts; or, cajole anyone to attend church?

By **telling his own story about his relationship to Jesus**, was this healed man *exposing* Jesus to the people, or *imposing* Jesus on the them?

Excurses:
Exposing vs. Evangelizing

Sitting in a hospital conference room, crowded with a wide spectrum of medical students, residents, and practicing medical professors, we'd gathered to hear a talk on Christian healthcare. The distinguished speaker gave a presentation filled with soaring philosophical ideas. Truthfully though, I don't recall one of them. What I do recall, and what is indelibly impressed in my memory, was the scrub-dressed doctor who stood up during the Q&A, weeping in front of us all, describing his sense of failure as a Christian in healthcare because he hadn't "evangelized many of my patients."

My heart broke and I began to weep, too. But not for the same reason as he. I wept for the failure of pastors and mentors to teach him what his responsibility really was. He was broken-hearted, not understanding that he was focusing on accomplishing a minor thing generally not appropriate to his vocation. And, He hadn't been trained to practice the major thing fitting for his setting. He fixated on evangelizing, rather than exposing Jesus, which was his main charge. To review Mark 4:1-34, your principal assignment as Christians in a healthcare setting is to sow, not cultivate, water, or reap.

This is not to say that as Christians you don't have the same Great Commission as all other Christians. You do. But if you read Matthew 28.18-20, the assignment is to baptize and teach the disciples (of Jesus) that you make. Making disciples first requires two key precursors: time (which is sorely lacking in your practice setting) and *that the person desire to become a follower of Jesus*. Who wants to become a follower of someone they don't know, have never heard of, or aren't sure is superior and worthy to be followed?

Exposing Jesus is something you can do each day and know you are fulfilling God's charge for your life and vocation. That's challenging and rewarding enough – **Psalm 126:5-6**.

Medicine Not Sufficient – Things You Can't Fix (Mark 5:24-34)

[24]{.sup} So Jesus went with him [Jairus, from v. 21-23], and a large crowd was following and pressing against Him. [25]{.sup} A woman suffering from bleeding for 12 years [26]{.sup} had endured much under many doctors. She had spent everything she had and was not helped at all. On the contrary, she became worse. [27]{.sup} Having heard about Jesus, she came behind Him in the crowd and touched His robe. [28]{.sup} For she said, "If I can just touch His robes, I'll be made well!" [29]{.sup} Instantly her flow of blood ceased, and she sensed in her body that she was cured of her affliction.

[30]{.sup} At once Jesus realized in Himself that power had gone out from Him. He turned around in the crowd and said, "Who touched My robes?"

[31]{.sup} His disciples said to Him, "You see the crowd pressing against You, and You say, 'Who touched Me?'"

[32]{.sup} So He was looking around to see who had done this. [33]{.sup} Then the woman, knowing what had happened to her, came with fear and trembling, fell down before Him, and told Him the whole truth. [34]{.sup} "Daughter," He said to her, "your faith has made you well. Go in peace and be free from your affliction."

Who exercised the faith sufficient to be healed?

From the human perspective, how did the woman come to have this faith (v.22)? Read **Romans 10:17** and **Isaiah 7:9b**.

From God's perspective, how did the woman get her faith and healing? Read **Ephesians 2:8**.

Curiously, you may have noticed that there is again no mention of what we, today, might label "the Gospel Message." The woman seemed to have put her faith in the person and work of Jesus, insofar as she knew Him from the testimony of others who had been healed. How does it make you feel to see God honor her 'incomplete' faith?

In this account, people served God and this woman by simply being witnesses of the person and work of Jesus in their lives. They moved her in the direction of healing.

Who actually healed the woman?

Where did the healing power come from?

What is your responsibility vis-à-vis God's? Read **Acts 1:7-8**.

Power Over Death Too – Christ Has All Power
(Mark 5:21-23, 35-43)

²¹ *When Jesus had crossed over again by boat to the other side, a large crowd gathered around Him while He was by the sea.* ²² *One of the synagogue leaders, named Jairus, came, and when he saw Jesus, he fell at His feet* ²³ *and kept begging Him, "My little daughter is at death's door. Come and lay Your hands on her so she can get well and live."*

---

³⁵ *While He was still speaking, people came from the synagogue leader's house and said, "Your daughter is dead. Why bother the Teacher anymore?"*

³⁶ *But when Jesus overheard what was said, He told the synagogue leader, "Don't be afraid. Only believe."* ³⁷ *He did not let anyone accompany Him except Peter, James, and John, James's brother.* ³⁸ *They came to the leader's house, and He saw a commotion—people weeping and wailing loudly.* ³⁹ *He went in and said to them, "Why are you making a commotion and weeping? The child is not dead but asleep."*

⁴⁰ *They started laughing at Him, but He put them all outside. He took the child's father, mother, and those who were with Him, and entered the place where the child was.* ⁴¹ *Then He took the child by the hand and said to her, "Talitha koum!" (which is translated, "Little girl, I say to you, get up!").* ⁴² *Immediately the girl got up and began to walk. (She was 12 years old.) At this they were utterly astounded.* ⁴³ *Then He gave them strict orders that no one should know about this and said that she should be given something to eat.*

Who exercised faith sufficient for the little girl to be healed?

Did everyone involved with the family, or with Jesus' circle of disciples, have to be involved or exercise faith in order for the little girl to be healed?

If you are curious why Jesus told the family and disciples to be quiet about the healing that had happened, especially in light of the things we've learned in this study, review the study on Mark 1:16-45.

Reflection

When speaking of Jesus and faith matters in the presence of a patient, peer, or employee, what does Jesus say are the two things you ought to talk about?

Speaking about what the Lord has done for you deals with how He has met your physical or soul needs, such as healing you or giving you wisdom. List two or three examples of what the Lord has done for you.

Speaking about the loving mercy God has had on you deals with your spiritual component. It shows how even in your sin God knew, loved, and redeemed you. You are no longer counted as guilty. You've been given eternal life and hope; indwelled by the Holy Spirit to help you live more like Jesus. Describe the loving mercy God has had on you.

Walking in Jesus' Footsteps Immediately

In spite of the example of the three amigos at the fiery furnace or the man born blind, there are enough examples of people not being healed/delivered, as you generally understand it, to make you guard against pressing the idea that faith always leads to temporal, physical healing.

As if to emphasize this point, Jesus prayed three times in the Garden of Gethsemane for deliverance but didn't receive it. Surely He prayed in faith.

Yet you have seen several times now that faith, whether that of a patient, or a concerned bystander, often plays a role in someone's healing.

Think on and write out what you believe is the biblical lesson about making faith a part of how you view your patients, and what role it will play in practicing Christian healthcare.

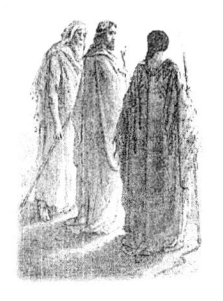

Mark 6

Tell Of Your Encounter With
The Omnipotent One (Part 2)

Mapping the Path Forward

Mark chapter six is the culmination of a major disciple-training period begun in chapter four and continued through chapter five. In chapter six, Jesus began passing to and through the disciples the responsibility of sharing the Lord's love and power with those who would listen and believe. He did so without sugarcoating or ambiguity, for it is made clear that just as Jesus was opposed, His disciples would be also.

This study has much to say to Christians in healthcare.

- Teach & tell your stories with God whether those you hope will listen do or don't.

- You have the same assignment to heal the body, teach the soul, and speak to the spirit that Jesus had in His incarnational ministry.

- Opposition to God may redound to you. You may be ignored, rejected, or have your livelihood threatened.

- The shepherd Moses cared about his flock, but Jesus – the Good Shepherd – is someone greater than Moses. You are the Good Shepherd's instrument of compassionate care.

- "Have courage. It is I. Don't be afraid."

- Faithfulness to telling your story with God leads to amazing change of hearts.

Rejected by His Hometown Friends and Family (Mark 6:1-6a)

6 ¹*He went away from there and came to His hometown, and His disciples followed Him.* ²*When the Sabbath came, He began to teach in the synagogue, and many who heard Him were astonished. "Where did this man get these things?" they said. "What is this wisdom given to Him, and how are these miracles performed by His hands?* ³*Isn't this the carpenter, the son of Mary, and the brother of James, Joses, Judas, and Simon? And aren't His sisters here with us?" So they were offended by Him.*

⁴*Then Jesus said to them, "A prophet is not without honor except in his hometown, among his relatives, and in his household."* ⁵*So He was not able to do any miracles there, except that He laid His hands on a few sick people and healed them.* ⁶*And He was amazed at their unbelief.*

Notice that Jesus healed, taught, and preached in the countryside (clinics), villages (hospitals) and in synagogues and the temple (the academic centers).

What is the key observation about the disciples you see in verse 1?

In the rest of this passage, the disciples were watching the interaction and the reactions of people to Jesus, and Jesus to the people. Now you, too, are observing.

What lessons do you take away from watching how Jesus responded to opposition and unbelief? Carefully consider and record how you see those lessons directly applying to opposition or unbelief coming from your administration, peers, coworkers, patients, or their families.

See One, Do One, Teach One
(Mark 6:6b-13)

Now He was going around the villages in a circuit, teaching. ⁷ He summoned the Twelve and began to send them out in pairs and gave them authority over unclean spirits. ⁸ He instructed them to take nothing for the road except a walking stick: no bread, no traveling bag, no money in their belts. ⁹ They were to wear sandals, but not put on an extra shirt. ¹⁰ Then He said to them, "Whenever you enter a house, stay there until you leave that place. ¹¹ If any place does not welcome you and people refuse to listen to you, when you leave there, shake the dust off your feet as a testimony against them."

¹² So they went out and preached that people should repent. ¹³ And they were driving out many demons, anointing many sick people with olive oil, and healing them.

Jesus and the disciples stayed within the region visiting and revisiting the same villages, seeing the same people over and over. How might this mode of operation apply to your healthcare setting and practice?

1. For the practitioner:

2. For the patients:

3. For those observing the practitioner interacting with patients:

Jesus had been healing bodies, teaching souls, and speaking to the spirits of the people. What part of Jesus' ministry did He assign to His disciples?

What might using olive oil represent for you today?

A Note Before You Move On

Remember that Jesus was still in the early stages of training His disciples. His followers were raised under the Law Moses brought, and the image of Moses as their shepherd and provider of manna from Heaven. The disciples were also living in a time when many were calling John the Baptist a prophet, maybe the one Moses had foretold would one day appear (Deuteronomy 18:15-19).

The next two accounts, Mark 6:14-29 and 6:30-44, are given, in part, to show that the age of the Law and the exclusively-human prophets has passed. Jesus has come as the Good Shepherd, the Bread of Life, sent from heaven. Jesus is the One foretold who would come to teach God's Word. Everything He says must be obeyed.

Don't be too harsh on the disciples not yet understanding what Jesus was doing and teaching. Every paradigm under which they had been raised was being replaced by a single person – Jesus.

The same goes for your patients. Have grace toward them when you say or suggest something that upends their worldview or sense of identity. Keep speaking the truth in love, with gentleness and respect. Allow them the space to reflect and question. Jesus didn't give up on the disciples. Neither should you give up on patients, if they are asking questions and considering your counsel.

On What Basis Do You Expect Earthly Justice? (Mark 6:14-29)

[14] *King Herod heard of this, because Jesus' name had become well known. Some said, "John the Baptist has been raised from the dead, and that's why supernatural powers are at work in him."* [15] *But others said, "He's Elijah." Still others said, "He's a prophet—like one of the prophets."*

[16] *When Herod heard of it, he said, "John, the one I beheaded, has been raised!"* [17] *For Herod himself had given orders to arrest John and to chain him in prison on account of Herodias, his brother Philip's wife, whom he had married.* [18] *John had been telling Herod, "It is not lawful for you to have your brother's wife!"* [19] *So Herodias held a grudge against him and wanted to kill him. But she could not,* [20] *because Herod was in awe of John and was protecting him, knowing he was a righteous and holy man. When Herod heard him he would be very disturbed, yet would hear him gladly.*

[21] *Now an opportune time came on his birthday, when Herod gave a banquet for his nobles, military commanders, and the leading men of Galilee.* [22] *When Herodias's own daughter came in and danced, she pleased Herod and his guests. The king said to the girl, "Ask me whatever you want, and I'll give it to you."* [23] *So he swore oaths to her: "Whatever you ask me I will give you, up to half my kingdom."*

[24] *Then she went out and said to her mother, "What should I ask for?"*

"John the Baptist's head!" she said.

[25] *Immediately she hurried to the king and said, "I want you to give me John the Baptist's head on a platter—right now!"*

²⁶ Though the king was deeply distressed, because of his oaths and the guests he did not want to refuse her. ²⁷ The king immediately sent for an executioner and commanded him to bring John's head. So he went and beheaded him in prison, ²⁸ brought his head on a platter, and gave it to the girl. Then the girl gave it to her mother. ²⁹ When his disciples heard about it, they came and removed his corpse and placed it in a tomb.

John the Baptist was the greatest prophet (**Luke** 7:24-28). Now, however, the time of prophets has passed.

History and experience show that not every follower of Jesus will face the kind of injustice John the Baptist faced. Are all disciples exempt from trouble and injustice though?

Read **John 16**. What provision has Jesus made for you when trouble comes?

With trouble, fear is usually not far away. **1 Peter 4:12-19** is great encouragement to hang on and hang in, despite persecution for Jesus' name. Why should being persecuted for being a Christian cause you to rejoice?

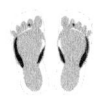

Give Your Little (Seed, Loaf, or Fish) to Jesus to Multiply
(Mark 6:30-44)

30 The apostles gathered around Jesus and reported to Him all that they had done and taught. 31 He said to them, "Come away by yourselves to a remote place and rest for a while." For many people were coming and going, and they did not even have time to eat. 32 So they went away in the boat by themselves to a remote place, 33 but many saw them leaving and recognized them. People ran there by land from all the towns and arrived ahead of them. 34 So as He stepped ashore, He saw a huge crowd and had compassion on them, because they were like sheep without a shepherd. Then He began to teach them many things.

35 When it was already late, His disciples approached Him and said, "This place is a wilderness, and it is already late! 36 Send them away, so they can go into the surrounding countryside and villages to buy themselves something to eat."

37 "You give them something to eat," He responded.

They said to Him, "Should we go and buy 200 denarii worth of bread and give them something to eat?"

38 And He asked them, "How many loaves do you have? Go look."

When they found out they said, "Five, and two fish."

39 Then He instructed them to have all the people sit down in groups on the green grass. 40 So they sat down in ranks of hundreds and fifties. 41 Then He took the five loaves and the two fish, and looking up to heaven, He blessed and broke the loaves. He kept giving them to His disciples to set before the people. He also divided the two fish among them all. 42 Everyone ate and was filled. 43 Then they picked up 12 baskets full of pieces of bread and fish. 44 Now those who ate the loaves were 5,000 men.

Moses brought the Law. Now the time of the Law has passed. **(Exodus 16:33; John 6)**

Verse 34 tells you Jesus had compassion on the people. Out of that compassion, what did Jesus *first* do for the people?

What does that say to you about the importance of being willing to speak truth, including both encouragement and admonition, hope, and your witness to a patient, coworker, or other person, when you feel compassion for them?

In the light of how Jesus ministers in this passage, are teaching your patients and others more godly ways of thinking, and meeting the physical needs of those for whom you feel compassion, either/or, or both/and responsibilities?

"Have Courage! It is I. Don't Be Afraid" (Mark 6:45-52)

[45] Immediately He made His disciples get into the boat and go ahead of Him to the other side, to Bethsaida, while He dismissed the crowd. [46] After He said good-bye to them, He went away to the mountain to pray. [47] When evening came, the boat was in the middle of the sea, and He was alone on the land. [48] He saw them being battered as they rowed because the wind was against them. Around three in the morning He came toward them walking on the sea and wanted to pass by them. [49] When they saw Him walking on the sea, they thought it was a ghost and cried out; [50] for they all saw Him and were terrified. Immediately He spoke with them and said, "Have courage! It is I. Don't be afraid." [51] Then He got into the boat with them, and the wind ceased. They were completely astounded,[1] [52] because they had not understood about the loaves. Instead, their hearts were hardened.

The expert fishermen had come to the end of their own knowledge and skill, to no avail. All during their efforts, struggles, and failure, Jesus probably could see them from the mountaintop as He prayed.

What lesson(s) do you think Jesus was trying to teach by waiting until about 3am to walk out to their boat and still the storm? Give particular attention to verses 51-52 as you formulate your answers.

Faithful Sowing Reaps a Huge Harvest for God (Mark 6:53-56)

⁵³ When they had crossed over, they came to land at Gennesaret and beached the boat. ⁵⁴ As they got out of the boat, people immediately recognized Him. ⁵⁵ They hurried throughout that vicinity and began to carry the sick on mats to wherever they heard He was. ⁵⁶ Wherever He would go, into villages, towns, or the country, they laid the sick in the market-places and begged Him that they might touch just the tassel of His robe. And everyone who touched it was made well.

Review **Mark 5:11-17** – How did the people react to Jesus healing the demon-possessed man and casting the demons into the pigs, which led to mass swine suicide and thousands of bobbing pork bellies on the Sea of Galilee?

Review **Mark 4:30-32** and **5:18-20** – On a relative scale, Jesus' assignment for the healed man was tiny. The man was simply to sow the mustard seeds of his personal witness of what the Lord had done for him and the loving mercy God had had on him. Was the healed man faithful to sow his small amount?

Apparently because of the healed man's faithfulness in the small things, what harvest was reaped in this passage?

Initially, friends and family rejected Jesus. Then they accepted Him. Will hometown friends and family always reject disciples of Jesus? If not, what does that tell you about being faithful to sow?

Reflection

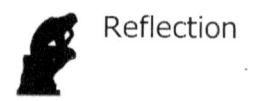

At this point in Jesus' incarnational ministry, He has come to the place where He assigns the disciples to go forth and do what He's been doing. The same assignment has come to you, too.

The disciples aren't perfect. They make mistakes and don't have full understanding, but God believes they have enough understanding to start walking like Him through the world.

Pause here and look back at this study and the ones that came before it. Of the many lessons you have completed, what key practices or ways of thinking have impacted you most? List three to five of them below.

Walking in Jesus' Footsteps Immediately

A crucial lesson of this chapter is the cyclical nature of Jesus' healthcare practice. He encourages sowing small seeds faithfully and regularly, and that includes sowing them over the same ground repeatedly.

In your practice, you will likely have many repeat visits from the same patients. Some will not be receptive to seed-sowing in early encounters, but over time, they may become receptive. That's between God and them. You are to sow.

Who do you know in your class, among your peers or co-workers, or your patients or their loved ones, to whom you may have said something exposing Jesus one time, and have never sown another seed? Maybe you let fear run you off the field as far as they are concerned. The point is Jesus has called you to keep sowing, for God is working in the background, in ways you know nothing about, to prepare formerly hard soil.

List at least one person you regularly see into whom you will commit to sow seed the next time you see him or her. The more people you list, the sooner you will be able to demonstrate faithfulness to your calling.

MARK 7

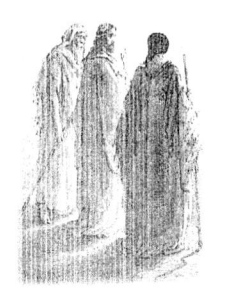

GOD KNOWS OUR HEARTS BUT DO WE?

Mapping the Path Forward

Mark seven challenges us to our core. Do you really worship God by your thoughts and actions or just play at it? Do you have ears to hear God speaking to you? Are you making right judgments about your patients, particularly whether they are worthy to have God intervene in their lives? Does God really do everything well, including helping both the figurative and literal deaf and dumb hear and praise Him? Are you willing to say so out loud?

What will this study have to say to Christians in healthcare?

- God is not a fan of hypocrisy. You must guard against it.

- Are you at risk of putting your rules over God's and thinking yourself godly?

- The Lord may very well test your worship, obedience, and faith by the people He brings into your path.

- He may also use you as His instrument to test the faith of others.

- Jesus expects His followers to speak up in praise of Him.

Religious Rules Deafen Us to God's Desires (Mark 7:1-23)

7 ¹ *The Pharisees and some of the scribes who had come from Jerusalem gathered around Him.* ² *They observed that some of His disciples were eating their bread with unclean—that is, unwashed—hands.* ³ *(For the Pharisees, in fact all the Jews, will not eat unless they wash their hands ritually, keeping the tradition of the elders.* ⁴ *When they come from the marketplace, they do not eat unless they have washed. And there are many other customs they have received and keep, like the washing of cups, jugs, copper utensils, and dining couches.)* ⁵ *Then the Pharisees and the scribes asked Him, "Why don't Your disciples live according to the tradition of the elders, instead of eating bread with ritually unclean hands?"*

⁶ *He answered them, "Isaiah prophesied correctly about you hypocrites, as it is written:*

These people honor Me with their lips,
but their heart is far from Me.
⁷ *They worship Me in vain,*
teaching as doctrines the commands of men.

⁸ *Disregarding the command of God, you keep the tradition of men."* ⁹ *He also said to them, "You completely invalidate God's command in order to maintain your tradition!* ¹⁰ *For Moses said:*

Honor your father and your mother; and
Whoever speaks evil of father or mother
must be put to death.

¹¹ *But you say, 'If a man tells his father or mother: Whatever benefit you might have received from me is Corban'" (that is, a gift committed to the temple),* ¹² *"you no longer let him do anything for his father or mother.* ¹³ *You revoke God's*

word by your tradition that you have handed down. And you do many other similar things." ¹⁴ *Summoning the crowd again, He told them, "Listen to Me, all of you, and understand:* ¹⁵ *Nothing that goes into a person from outside can defile him, but the things that come out of a person are what defile him. [*¹⁶ *If anyone has ears to hear, he should listen!]"*

¹⁷ *When He went into the house away from the crowd, the disciples asked Him about the parable.* ¹⁸ *And He said to them, "Are you also as lacking in understanding? Don't you realize that nothing going into a man from the outside can defile him?* ¹⁹ *For it doesn't go into his heart but into the stomach and is eliminated." (As a result, He made all foods clean.)* ²⁰ *Then He said, "What comes out of a person—that defiles him.* ²¹ *For from within, out of people's hearts, come evil thoughts, sexual immoralities, thefts, murders,* ²² *adulteries, greed, evil actions, deceit, promiscuity, stinginess, blasphemy, pride, and foolishness.* ²³ *All these evil things come from within and defile a person."*

What are some of the nice labels for optional behaviors which serve as social lubricant and markers of cultural identity?

R_____, C_____, and T_____.

Jesus and Isaiah warn nice labels can become whitewash for D_____ and C_____, meaning they are no longer considered optional, but demand strict observance. Disobedience leads to punishment and/or ostracism.

Using an example in verses 8-15, Jesus warns of what danger, once optional behaviors become rigid expectations – label creep?

Give examples of how label creep can become a part of your medical practice. To get you thinking, label creep could impact social norms, administrative standards, or medical guidelines.

Over centuries and across the languages of Hebrew, Greek, and English, 'heart,' 'mind,' and 'soul' have become somewhat synonymous. How do you guard against defiling your soul?

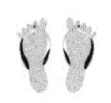

The "Dog" Would Not Be Dumb About Her Faith (Mark 7:24-30)

[24] *He got up and departed from there to the region of Tyre and Sidon. He entered a house and did not want anyone to know it, but He could not escape notice.* [25] *Instead, immediately after hearing about Him, a woman whose little daughter had an unclean spirit came and fell at His feet.* [26] *Now the woman was Greek, a Syrophoenician by birth, and she kept asking Him to drive the demon out of her daughter.* [27] *He said to her, "Allow the children to be satisfied first, because it isn't right to take the children's bread and throw it to the dogs."*

[28] *But she replied to Him, "Lord, even the dogs under the table eat the children's crumbs."*

[29] *Then He told her, "Because of this reply, you may go. The demon has gone out of your daughter."* [30] *When she went back to her home, she found her child lying on the bed, and the demon was gone.*

To make His point in a physical sense, Jesus left Israel and went to the land of the Gentiles – the 'dogs.' This was despite His declaration that His mission was to the children of Israel.

Is uncleanness a result of gender, race, religion, socio-economics or any other feature of circumstance?

How did Jesus test the woman's faith (verse 27)?

How did the woman prove her faith?

Do you have faith such as this woman's?

Why or why not?

How has your faith been tested and proved? Take time to reflect upon your answer here, because how you answer may well find its way into a discussion with someone who needs their faith strengthened.

If you have ever looked at a patient, or read their medical record, and presumed they were incapable of such faith because of their appearance or behavior, how does this account change the way you'll look at their faith, or potential faith, in the future?

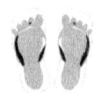

Jesus Does All Things Well, Including Saving the Deaf & Dumb (Mark 7:31-37)

³¹ Again, leaving the region of Tyre, He went by way of Sidon to the Sea of Galilee, through the region of the Decapolis. ³² They brought to Him a deaf man who also had a speech difficulty, and begged Jesus to lay His hand on him. ³³ So He took him away from the crowd privately. After putting His fingers in the man's ears and spitting, He touched his tongue. ³⁴ Then, looking up to heaven, He sighed deeply and said to him, "Ephphatha!" (that is, "Be opened!"). ³⁵ Immediately his ears were opened, his speech difficulty was removed, and he began to speak clearly. ³⁶ Then He ordered them to tell no one, but the more He would order them, the more they would proclaim it.

³⁷ They were extremely astonished and said, "He has done everything well! He even makes deaf people hear, and people unable to speak, talk!"

What do you think the spiritual lesson is of this encounter? (Hint: In the first vignette, the religious rulers were deaf to the things of God; in the second, the woman refused to be dumb about her faith.) How then would this encounter sum it up?

Read **Mark 7:36, Luke 2:13-14,** and **19:37-40**. At each end of Jesus' incarnational ministry, God's followers, be they angelic or human, were willing to come down from their heights to proclaim glory to God. Only those who thought highly of themselves or their man-made doctrines and commands insisted on silence rather than praise. Since Jesus knew the rocks would cry out His glory in the face of silence, surely He didn't expect that the healed man and the witnesses who were astonished by Him would actually be quiet. Rather, this sign of healing the deaf and dumb man seems to be a statement to, in a sense, shame those who are free to give God praise and yet refuse to speak up.

In what way does this account of a deaf and dumb person whom God healed alter or strengthen how you see your responsibility to God and toward your patients as a Christian practicing healthcare?

Reflection

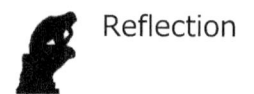

It is important to take away from this lesson three points about making judgments regarding other people and their behavior.

1. You are not their judge unto eternal life – God is. Therefore, you are not to be judgmental in the sense of thinking someone is not worthy of God's love or salvation (Luke 6:37).

2. You are called to make a right judgment about what God wants for a person (John 7:21-24). That means thinking about another person using God's righteous standards, not your own.

3. You are to judge a person's actions as a fruit inspector (Matthew 7:15-20). This is part of discernment and good shepherding.

If there is a person or group of people you previously wrote off as unworthy of salvation because they don't live up to your doctrines or commands, note them here. There is transformational power in writing down their names.

Walking in Jesus' Footsteps Immediately

If you wrote down the name of a person or group of people you've written off in your classroom or workplace, good. Now don't go any further until you pray about it. Confess and repent that you've put your doctrines and commands ahead of God's desire that none should perish.

What has God told you to do to make amends and follow Him?

Go do it.

Mark 8

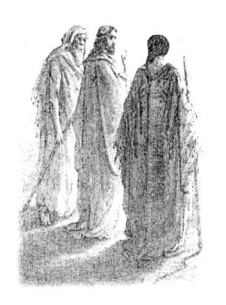

Spiritual Vision

Mapping the Path Forward

Mark eight is about seeing with spiritual eyes – your need to see the world as God sees it. There are times when the only vision that will lead to healing is spiritual.

For insight into events in Mark 8, let's review a few points about Bethsaida, which features prominently. The name Bethsaida means house or place of fishing/hunting. It is the place from which Peter, Philip, and Andrew came, and where they may have attended the religious school attached to the synagogue. These men were called out of Bethsaida to become fishers of people. It is also where they withdrew immediately after feeding 5,000 men plus women and children with five loaves and two fish. They rowed unsuccessfully all night to get to Bethsaida; Jesus nearly walked by the boat when they saw Him as a ghost rather than the Lord. Jesus also condemned Bethsaida for unwillingness to believe His message, even though He did many miracles there.

This study says much to Christians in healthcare.?

- Persistently looking at only your own resources to do God's work is a sign of poor spiritual eyesight. It's fair to say Jesus finds this highly annoying.

- Ditto for forgetting (not seeing) the works God has done for you in the past and not letting these build your faith for future needs.

- When you see that someone has a blind spot to behavior that is detrimental to self or others, it is not sin to point that out as part of teaching a soul.

- Developing spiritual vision requires that you focus on where God is going and what He is doing, rather than blindly following man's thoughts and ways.

Don't You See Yet?
(Mark 8:1-21)

8 ¹*In those days there was again a large crowd, and they had nothing to eat. He summoned the disciples and said to them,* ²*"I have compassion on the crowd, because they've already stayed with Me three days and have nothing to eat.* ³*If I send them home hungry they will collapse on the way, and some of them have come a long distance."*

⁴ *His disciples answered Him, "Where can anyone get enough bread here in this desolate place to fill these people?"*

⁵ *"How many loaves do you have?" He asked them.*

"Seven," they said. ⁶ *Then He commanded the crowd to sit down on the ground. Taking the seven loaves, He gave thanks, broke the loaves, and kept on giving them to His disciples to set before the people. So they served the loaves to the crowd.* ⁷ *They also had a few small fish, and when He had blessed them, He said these were to be served as well.* ⁸ *They ate and were filled. Then they collected seven large baskets of leftover pieces.* ⁹ *About 4,000 men were there. He dismissed them* ¹⁰ *and immediately got into the boat with His disciples and went to the district of Dalmanutha.*

¹¹ *The Pharisees came out and began to argue with Him, demanding of Him a sign from heaven to test Him.* ¹² *But sighing deeply in His spirit, He said, "Why does this generation demand a sign? I assure you: No sign will be given to this generation!"* ¹³ *Then He left them, got on board the boat again, and went to the other side.*

¹⁴ *They had forgotten to take bread and had only one loaf with them in the boat.* ¹⁵ *Then He commanded them: "Watch out! Beware of the yeast of the Pharisees and the yeast of Herod."*

[16] They were discussing among themselves that they did not have any bread. [17] Aware of this, He said to them, "Why are you discussing that you do not have any bread? Don't you understand or comprehend? Is your heart hardened? [18] Do you have eyes, and not see, and do you have ears, and not hear? And do you not remember? [19] When I broke the five loaves for the 5,000, how many baskets full of pieces of bread did you collect?"

"Twelve," they told Him.

[20] "When I broke the seven loaves for the 4,000, how many large baskets full of pieces of bread did you collect?"

"Seven," they said.

[21] And He said to them, "Don't you understand yet?"

Looking at verse 3, what is Jesus' driving motivation?

Whom was Jesus compassionate toward?

Why them, possibly as opposed to all hungry people?

Were the disciples using fleshly or spiritual eyes in verse 4?

Read John chapter 6, if you have time. Recall that a sign is a physical object or event viewed as teaching a spiritual lesson.

What made Jesus sigh, in verses Mark 8:11-12?

What was Jesus chastising the disciples for in verses 13-21?

Describe how this can creep into how you practice medicine.

Seeing Spit as a Sign of Growing Spiritual Vision (Mark 8:22-26)

²² Then they came to Bethsaida. They brought a blind man to Him and begged Him to touch him. ²³ He took the blind man by the hand and brought him out of the village. Spitting on his eyes and laying His hands on him, He asked him, "Do you see anything?"

²⁴ He looked up and said, "I see people—they look to me like trees walking."

²⁵ Again Jesus placed His hands on the man's eyes, and he saw distinctly. He was cured and could see everything clearly. ²⁶ Then He sent him home, saying, "Don't even go into the village."

As a sign, Jesus used spittle in the eyes of the man of Bethsaida to restore his sight. Spit was thought by some Jews to have medicinal value. Jesus used His spit to heal at least three people. However, spitting on someone was also a sign of disdain and scorn in this culture. In addition, Jewish culture considered debilitations such as blindness a punishment from God in retribution for sin.

Use your own spiritual eyes now. Think carefully about the lessons of spiritual vision this story might be here to teach us.

Was the man born or did he become blind? There's a clue.

Jesus had healed many in and around Bethsaida. Yet only now the disciples bring the blind man to Him. Speculate why the disciples acted now, and what it suggests about their own developing spiritual vision.

What does it say to you, as a disciple of Jesus yourself, that the disciples brought the man out of Bethsaida to Jesus before Jesus applied spit to miraculously heal him?

What might it mean that Jesus told the spit-healed man not to return to Bethsaida?

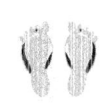

The Key to Seeing with Spiritual Eyes
(Mark 8:27-30)

²⁷ *Jesus went out with His disciples to the villages of Caesarea Philippi. And on the road He asked His disciples, "Who do people say that I am?"*

²⁸ *They answered Him, "John the Baptist; others, Elijah; still others, one of the prophets."*

²⁹ *"But you," He asked them again, "who do you say that I am?"*

Peter answered Him, "You are the Messiah!"

³⁰ *And He strictly warned them to tell no one about Him.*

-----

¹³ *When Jesus came to the region of Caesarea Philippi, He asked His disciples, "Who do people say that the Son of Man is?"*

¹⁴ *And they said, "Some say John the Baptist; others, Elijah; still others, Jeremiah or one of the prophets."*

¹⁵ *"But you," He asked them, "who do you say that I am?"*

¹⁶ *Simon Peter answered, "You are the Messiah, the Son of the living God!"*

¹⁷ *And Jesus responded, "Simon son of Jonah, you are blessed because flesh and blood did not reveal this to you, but My Father in heaven.*

Matthew 16:13-17

Jesus used the statements of other people to demonstrate that most people look at the person and work of Jesus based upon what they can see with their eyes of flesh. So they misidentify who He really is and why he came.

Is that the same habit the disciples had?

From Matthew's account, how did Jesus reveal that bad habit would be broken and a new one begun?

Do you believe that God the Father wants to reveal things to you – His child and His ambassador of reconciliation – too?

If so, in what ways might God give you spiritual insights? If not, why?

Be Careful Whose Eyes You Use
(Mark 8:31-33)

³¹ Then He began to teach them that the Son of Man must suffer many things and be rejected by the elders, the chief priests, and the scribes, be killed, and rise after three days. ³² He was openly talking about this. So Peter took Him aside and began to rebuke Him.

³³ But turning around and looking at His disciples, He rebuked Peter and said, "Get behind Me, Satan, because you're not thinking about God's concerns, but man's!"

There are three ways to look at things:

- M_____'s,
- S_____'s, and
- G_____'s.

A friend asks you how they can tell the difference between seeing things man's way, Satan's way, and God's way. What would you tell them are some distinguishing marks of each?

Man's View:

Satan's View:

God's View:

How might you prepare to see things from God's viewpoint?

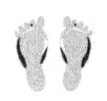

Spiritual Eyes See in Four Dimensions
(Mark 8:34-38)

³⁴ *Summoning the crowd along with His disciples, He said to them, "If anyone wants to be My follower, he must deny himself, take up his cross, and follow Me. ³⁵ For whoever wants to save his life will lose it, but whoever loses his life because of Me and the gospel will save it. ³⁶ For what does it benefit a man to gain the whole world yet lose his life? ³⁷ What can a man give in exchange for his life? ³⁸ For whoever is ashamed of Me and of My words in this adulterous and sinful generation, the Son of Man will also be ashamed of him when He comes in the glory of His Father with the holy angels."*

If your physical eyes are healthy, you see things in three dimensions: along a +/- x, a +/- y, and a +/- z axis.

However, you live in a world of at least four dimensions. Curiously, in this world the fourth dimension has only a positive axis. You call what would be its negative axis 'memories.' Even more challenging for you to comprehend, the fourth dimension doesn't exist in heaven or hell.

What is the fourth dimension?

How does this fourth dimension enter into how you see things spiritually? If you are not sure how to answer the question, reread the passage and ask yourself what point Jesus is trying to make.

Reflection

Write a definition of what it means to have spiritual vision.

Describe how you see spiritual vision integrating into the way you will provide Christian healthcare. Give consideration to how it affects your view of health, your interactions with patients and peers, etc., and seeing yourself as an agent of grace and an ambassador of reconciliation.

Walking in Jesus' Footsteps Immediately

Pray now, asking God if there is any area of your life, including your healthcare practice, where Satan controls how you see things. Ask God to deliver you from Satan's bondage to his viewpoint.

Write down what God revealed and how you will cooperate with Him for deliverance.

Repeat the process for any area God reveals you are looking at your healthcare practice according to mankind's standards, rather than from God's point-of-view.

Mark 9

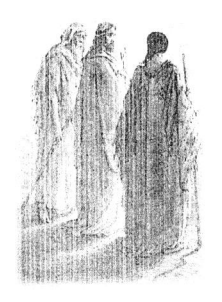

Christian Healthcare Must Be Bound To Jesus

Mapping the Path Forward

Jesus expands on spiritual vision – to see things the way God sees them, not only now, but as they could be in the future. God challenges disciples: look at things of the past as pointing to the present; the present is not what it appears; and, if you don't look at who you are and ought to be in Jesus, you will never be the disciple He desires you to be. Do you have eyes to see – really see – how this will affect your healthcare ministry?

What will this study have to say to Christians in healthcare?

- When guilt afflicts a patient, the Law and the Prophets are there to confirm they have sinned against God and are guilty. They need to be saved from God's wrath and condemnation. The Good News is Jesus the Savior has come, so they can be free of condemnation and live under grace, if they believe and choose to.

- As a Christian in healthcare, following Jesus means being willing to personally invest in some of your patients.

- No matter how intellectual you are, you must be able to communicate the Good News of Jesus understandably.

- You must be an excellent practitioner for a host of reasons, but you must trust Jesus to do the true healing.

- If you are going to remain salty, you must be willing to put off the sin that so easily entangles you. Do you seek personal healing from Jesus?

The Kingdom of God
(Mark 8:31-9:1)

⁸:³¹ Then He began to teach them that the Son of Man must suffer many things and be rejected by the elders, the chief priests, and the scribes, be killed, and rise after three days. ³² He was openly talking about this. So Peter took Him aside and began to rebuke Him.

³³ But turning around and looking at His disciples, He rebuked Peter and said, "Get behind Me, Satan, because you're not thinking about God's concerns, but man's!"

³⁴ Summoning the crowd along with His disciples, He said to them, "If anyone wants to be My follower, he must deny himself, take up his cross, and follow Me. ³⁵ For whoever wants to save his life will lose it, but whoever loses his life because of Me and the gospel will save it. ³⁶ For what does it benefit a man to gain the whole world yet lose his life? ³⁷ What can a man give in exchange for his life? ³⁸ For whoever is ashamed of Me and of My words in this adulterous and sinful generation, the Son of Man will also be ashamed of him when He comes in the glory of His Father with the holy angels."

9 ¹Then He said to them, "I assure you: There are some standing here who will not taste death until they see the kingdom of God come in power."

With great sternness, frankness, and authority, Jesus declares in verses 31-33 that God's concern is the d_____, b_____, and r_____ of the Son of Man. (This includes having an understanding of the purpose and meaning of these things.) This is broadly known to us as the G_____, meaning Good News.

Jesus spoke verse 34a to whom?

Jesus forthrightly declared in verses 34b-35 what it will take to be a subject in His kingdom. What are the requirements for citizenship in the kingdom of God?

While this life is important, Jesus is primarily teaching in verses 36-38 that disciples must have spiritual vision, spiritual hearing, and a spiritual voice. Having spiritual vision means focusing on eternity. Having spiritual hearing means to follow the Holy Spirit's leading, including listening for the spiritual concerns patients and peers raise. A spiritual voice is one that sows spiritual seeds and shares the Good News about the loving person and work of Jesus.

In verse 9:1, Jesus speaks again of God's kingdom. Recall a kingdom has a king who is a rightful heir to the throne, a throne, a place over which he has dominion, and subjects loyal to him. Previously you learned that the kingdom of God is n_____ to your patients or peers if two circumstances exist:

1. Jesus sits on the throne of your heart. He is your King, and as His loyal subject, He has indwelled you with the Holy Spirit. That makes you His ambassador of reconciliation.

2. You enter into the presence of a patient or peer, willing to serve your King as His ambassador to that person.

The kingdom of God will come in power when Jesus returns to take His loyal subjects to heaven, their eternal home. The next module is a glimpse of what that will be like.

1 Corinthians 15:42-26 and **1 Thessalonians 1:5-6** give many additional details about what it will be like when Jesus comes in power. Detail the events, sights, and sounds, etc. that will let everyone know Jesus has returned in power for His own.

Sharing details like these gave great comfort to my dying father, David, as I sat night vigil with him during his final two weeks. How might speaking about these details give hope to those you might care for or work with?

Law & Prophets Replaced by Covenant of Grace in Christ
(Mark 9:2-13)

² After six days Jesus took Peter, James, and John and led them up on a high mountain by themselves to be alone. He was transformed in front of them, ³ and His clothes became dazzling—extremely white as no launderer on earth could whiten them. ⁴ Elijah appeared to them with Moses, and they were talking with Jesus.

⁵ Then Peter said to Jesus, "Rabbi, it's good for us to be here! Let us make three tabernacles: one for You, one for Moses, and one for Elijah"— ⁶ because he did not know what he should say, since they were terrified.

⁷ A cloud appeared, overshadowing them, and a voice came from the cloud:

This is My beloved Son;
listen to Him!

⁸ Then suddenly, looking around, they no longer saw anyone with them except Jesus alone.

⁹ As they were coming down from the mountain, He ordered them to tell no one what they had seen until the Son of Man had risen from the dead. ¹⁰ They kept this word to themselves, discussing what "rising from the dead" meant.

¹¹ Then they began to question Him, "Why do the scribes say that Elijah must come first?"

¹² "Elijah does come first and restores everything," He replied. "How then is it written about the Son of Man that He must suffer many things and be treated with contempt? ¹³ But I tell you that Elijah really has come, and they did whatever they pleased to him, just as it is written about him."

About *transfigure* and *transform*. Depending upon the English translation, you may read Jesus was transfigured or transformed on the mountain, in front of the three amigos. Though in English the words are sometimes used interchangeably, for they have some overlapping features, they are not in a strict sense one-to-one synonyms. *Transfigure* means to in some way alter the external appearance of something, maybe to glorify or exalt it. The object appears different but remains recognizable from its prior appearance. Think of a lightbulb's appearance when off and then when turned on, or your dog after it has been to the groomer. *Transform* means to so alter the state of something as to make it essentially unrecognizable from its original state. Something new has been created. Think of a caterpillar becoming a butterfly. Renewing your mind – having the mind of Christ – should, through the lifelong process of sanctification, transform your life and conduct into the likeness of Christ.

In verses 2-10, seeing with fleshly eyes again, leads to not seeing the sign – not grasping the spiritual message – behind the appearance of Moses and Elijah. So God, in effect, blinds the disciples so they can't use their fleshly vision. Give an example of a time you first saw something from a fleshly viewpoint, only later recognizing it was a sign with a spiritual message.

For a deeper understanding of what Jesus was saying about Elijah, see Malachi 4:4-6; and Matthew 11:11-15, 17:10-13. The concept of Jesus as the suffering Son of Man is expressed in Psalm 22 and Isaiah 52:13-53:12.

Excurses:
Overshadowing

The concept of 'overshadowing' appears in Genesis 1:2, in Luke 1:34-35, and in Mark 9:2-10. Each time, the old way of things begins to be transformed and new creation occurs.

In Genesis, what transformed and what new creation appeared?

At the overshadowing in Luke, what transformation began and what new creation appeared?

Read **2 Peter 1:16-21, Acts 2:1-40**, and **2 Corinthians 5:16-21**. At the overshadowing in Mark, what transformation began and what new creation began appearing?

Read **Acts 5:12-16** and **2 Corinthians. 5:13-21**. If the Holy Spirit indwells you, and He overshadows, how might cooperating with Him impact your patients and coworkers?

I Do Believe-ish
(Mark 9:14-29)

14 When they came to the disciples, they saw a large crowd around them and scribes disputing with them. 15 All of a sudden, when the whole crowd saw Him, they were amazed and ran to greet Him. 16 Then He asked them, "What are you arguing with them about?"

17 Out of the crowd, one man answered Him, "Teacher, I brought my son to You. He has a spirit that makes him unable to speak. 18 Wherever it seizes him, it throws him down, and he foams at the mouth, grinds his teeth, and becomes rigid. So I asked Your disciples to drive it out, but they couldn't."

19 He replied to them, "You unbelieving generation! How long will I be with you? How long must I put up with you? Bring him to Me." 20 So they brought him to Him. When the spirit saw Him, it immediately convulsed the boy. He fell to the ground and rolled around, foaming at the mouth. 21 "How long has this been happening to him?" Jesus asked his father.

"From childhood," he said. 22 "And many times it has thrown him into fire or water to destroy him. But if You can do anything, have compassion on us and help us."

23 Then Jesus said to him, "'If You can'? Everything is possible to the one who believes."

24 Immediately the father of the boy cried out, "I do believe! Help my unbelief."

25 When Jesus saw that a crowd was rapidly coming together, He rebuked the unclean spirit, saying to it, "You mute and deaf spirit, I command you: come out of him and never enter him again!"

²⁶ Then it came out, shrieking and convulsing him violently. The boy became like a corpse, so that many said, "He's dead." ²⁷ But Jesus, taking him by the hand, raised him, and he stood up.

²⁸ After He went into a house, His disciples asked Him privately, "Why couldn't we drive it out?"

²⁹ And He told them, "This kind can come out by nothing but prayer [and fasting]."

Right after the transfiguration, the people seeing Jesus were 'amazed.' Why? (Possible hints are found in Exodus 34:29-35; 2 Corinthians 3:7-18; Hebrews 1:3.)

The challenge to the disciples in verses 16-27 leads to the question: In your healthcare ministry, where will your faith be focused – on your own skills and knowledge, or on God's compassion and power?

Are you willing to invest yourself, as Jesus said to in verses 28-29, in some of your patients? If not, why?

Consider the following to be a model of how to do that kind of investing in patients with difficult problems:

1. In faith pray earnestly and persistently.

2. Call upon the name of Jesus of Nazareth.

3. If no answer appears, add fasting to your earnest, persistent prayer.

4. If the answer to what you prayed for remains "No," it doesn't mean your faith or God failed, but that you were being given a chance to prove your faith by asking and trusting God no matter the answer.

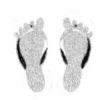

Grasp and Share the Gospel & Its Meaning (Mark 9:30-32)

³⁰ Then they left that place and made their way through Galilee, but He did not want anyone to know it. ³¹ For He was teaching His disciples and telling them, "The Son of Man is being betrayed into the hands of men. They will kill Him, and after He is killed, He will rise three days later." ³² But they did not understand this statement, and they were afraid to ask Him.

What are the essentials Jesus wants His disciples to grasp and tell?

Sin: We all do it and, thus, need a Savior.

Jesus: The sinless God-man who paid God's penalty for anyone who will accept it. He did it because God loves us and wants an eternal relationship with us.

His Death: The cost of God's wrath against sin.

Burial: Proof He was dead and exemplifying His separation from God, having taken on the sin of the world.

Resurrection: God raised Jesus for two reasons. First, to show He accepted the penalty Jesus paid. Second, to demonstrate He has the power He said He had to raise His followers glorified, immortal, and incorruptible too.

It's About the Power in Jesus' Name
(Mark 9:33-41)

[33] *Then they came to Capernaum. When He was in the house, He asked them, "What were you arguing about on the way?"* [34] *But they were silent, because on the way they had been arguing with one another about who was the greatest.* [35] *Sitting down, He called the Twelve and said to them, "If anyone wants to be first, he must be last of all and servant of all."* [36] *Then He took a child, had him stand among them, and taking him in His arms, He said to them,* [37] *"Whoever welcomes one little child such as this in My name welcomes Me. And whoever welcomes Me does not welcome Me, but Him who sent Me."*

[38] *John said to Him, "Teacher, we saw someone driving out demons in Your name, and we tried to stop him because he wasn't following us."*

[39] *"Don't stop him," said Jesus, "because there is no one who will perform a miracle in My name who can soon afterward speak evil of Me.* [40] *For whoever is not against us is for us.* [41] *And whoever gives you a cup of water to drink because of My name, since you belong to the Messiah—I assure you: He will never lose his reward.*

In whose name do you practice Christian healthcare?

Where is the power for healing really found?

Read the passage carefully. What are your responsibilities when it comes to how you use the gifts God has given you to practice medicine?

Heal Thyself First
(Mark 9:42-50)

⁴² "But whoever causes the downfall of one of these little ones who believe in Me—it would be better for him if a heavy millstone were hung around his neck and he were thrown into the sea. ⁴³ And if your hand causes your downfall, cut it off. It is better for you to enter life maimed than to have two hands and go to hell—the unquenchable fire, [⁴⁴ where

Their worm does not die,
and the fire is not quenched.]

⁴⁵ And if your foot causes your downfall, cut it off. It is better for you to enter life lame than to have two feet and be thrown into hell— [the unquenchable fire, ⁴⁶ where

Their worm does not die,
and the fire is not quenched.]

⁴⁷ And if your eye causes your downfall, gouge it out. It is better for you to enter the kingdom of God with one eye than to have two eyes and be thrown into hell, ⁴⁸ where

Their worm does not die,
and the fire is not quenched.

⁴⁹ For everyone will be salted with fire. ⁵⁰ Salt is good, but if the salt should lose its flavor, how can you make it salty? Have salt among yourselves and be at peace with one another."

The use of salt and fire symbolizes the total sacrifice of a burnt offering a Jew would make to God. In Romans 12:1, Jesus calls all of His followers to be given over totally to His rule and plans as a spiritual act of worship.

In this passage, how often does Jesus tell the disciples to be judgmental toward others?

How frequently does He tell disciples to judge themselves?

Why do you think Jesus called upon the disciples to judge themselves and 'get right' before He talked about being salty?

What are some situations in your practice which prime you to be judgmental of others – that cause you to use salty language in a worldly sense but not the spiritual sense?

Reflection

Which of these passages resonated the most with you? Why?

How will what you learned from this passage improve the way you provide Christian healthcare to your patients?

In what way does seeing how closely you must be bound to Jesus alter the way you understand what Christian healthcare really means?

Walking in Jesus' Footsteps Immediately

In healthcare you are constantly engaging with people having struggles. They may be patients, peers, or loved ones. Almost certainly at least one of these people has a problem that you haven't successfully 'fixed' using good medicine or sound teaching practices alone.

Write down the initials of one or more of these people. Describe their intractable issue in a few words.

Journal here how you pray and fast, seeking their healing.

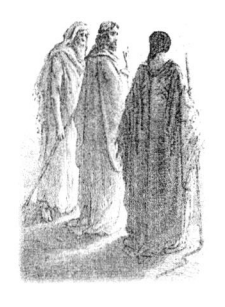

Mark 10

God's Plan For Healing Relationships

Mapping the Path Forward

For Christians in healthcare, Mark 10 is about discovering God's plan for how you study and practice in your privileged position. Look at the passages and glean from them principles for God-honoring attitudes such as putting God first, sacrifice, and humility. Consider how you will put these attitudes into practice.

Here are some things this study says to Christians in healthcare:

- Along with healing bodies and speaking to spirits, teaching souls is one of the three critical aspects of Christian healthcare. Teaching should always occur with gentleness and respect and consistently have at its core God's intentions and truth, even if you are righteously indignant over destructive or obstructive behavior.

- Loving the Lord God with all of your heart, soul, mind, and strength means being willing to take up your cross daily in His service. It also means that you devote the time, talents, and treasure He has given you to His service. You sow the seeds He has given you for His harvest. He promises He will not only produce a harvest 30, 60 or 100 fold, but give you bread to eat *and* more seeds to sow.

- Loving God, He promises, will also result in persecutions. You must train yourself to endure and overcome them.

- You may in fact be the smartest, most highly educated and compensated person in any room. SO WHAT!? God is looking for humility. A humble and contrite heart He will not despise. An arrogant attitude is the path to a fall.

Teaching People to Fulfill God's Plan (Mark 10:1-16)

10 ¹*He set out from there and went to the region of Judea and across the Jordan. Then crowds converged on Him again and, as He usually did, He began teaching them once more.* ²*Some Pharisees approached Him to test Him. They asked, "Is it lawful for a man to divorce his wife?"*

³*He replied to them, "What did Moses command you?"*

⁴*They said, "Moses permitted us to write divorce papers and send her away."*

⁵*But Jesus told them, "He wrote this command for you because of the hardness of your hearts.* ⁶*But from the beginning of creation God made them male and female.*

⁷*For this reason a man will leave his father and mother [and be joined to his wife],*
⁸*and the two will become one flesh.*

So they are no longer two, but one flesh. ⁹*Therefore what God has joined together, man must not separate."*

¹⁰*Now in the house the disciples questioned Him again about this matter.* ¹¹*And He said to them, "Whoever divorces his wife and marries another commits adultery against her.* ¹²*Also, if she divorces her husband and marries another, she commits adultery."*

¹³*Some people were bringing little children to Him so He might touch them, but His disciples rebuked them.* ¹⁴*When Jesus saw it, He was indignant and said to them, "Let the little children come to Me. Don't stop them, for the kingdom of God belongs to such as these.* ¹⁵*I assure you: Whoever does not welcome the kingdom of God like a little child will never enter it."* ¹⁶*After taking them in His arms, He laid His hands on them and blessed them.*

In the first 12 verses, the Pharisees seemed to be asking Jesus to condone sin. What was Jesus' response?

Whose intentions and standards are the benchmarks Jesus uses?

Considering God's intentions and standards, list at least three reasons why Jesus would be opposed to a family breaking up.

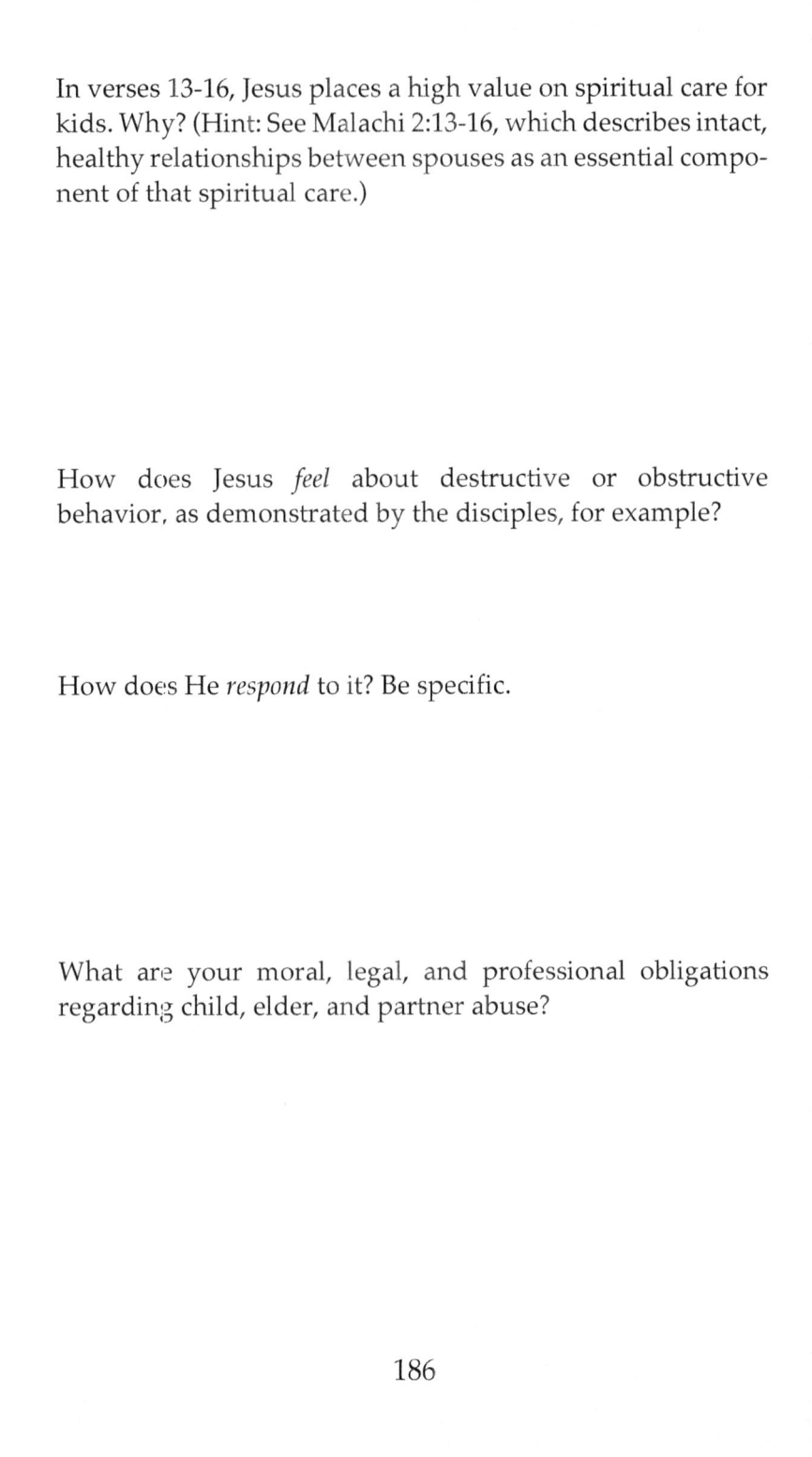

In verses 13-16, Jesus places a high value on spiritual care for kids. Why? (Hint: See Malachi 2:13-16, which describes intact, healthy relationships between spouses as an essential component of that spiritual care.)

How does Jesus *feel* about destructive or obstructive behavior, as demonstrated by the disciples, for example?

How does He *respond* to it? Be specific.

What are your moral, legal, and professional obligations regarding child, elder, and partner abuse?

Excurses:
Divorce and the Meaning of Adultery

As a paramedic, I saw emotional, physical, financial, and social shrapnel wounds of exploded marriages. As a pastor, I dealt with ugly, debilitating spiritual scars left behind long after the court battles ended. Faced with caring for the wounded, I had to delve deeply into the issue of divorce. Since the only ground Jesus gave for it was adultery (Gr. *Porneia*), I needed to try to understand what He meant by the word.

After studying Jewish, Roman Catholic, and protestant scholars, I concluded the following definition is a sound explanation of adultery, as used in Scripture:

> "Biblically-recognized abandonment, violence, sexual covetousness, or sexual immorality which one spouse commits against the other, compromising God's intended unity, sanctity, or privilege in marriage."

If you wish to delve into the Scriptures for your own edification and preparation to teach and speak to patients or peers, I recommend using The Amplified Bible (Grand Rapids, Zondervan, 1987) to examine Scripture passages about the following sins.

Abandonment:
Exodus 21:10-11, Genesis 1:27-28c, 1 Corinthians 7:1-16

Violence:
Malachi 2:13-16, Ephesians 5:28-31

Sexual Covetousness:
Genesis 9:22-23, Exodus 20:26, Matthew 5:27-28

Sexual Immorality:
Leviticus 18:6-20, Matthew 5, 1 Corinthians 7, Hebrews 13:4

This definition is only part of divorce counseling. Among many things, you must also talk about repentance and forgiveness.

Using Your Possessions to Facilitate God's Plan (Mark 10:17-31)

[17] *As He was setting out on a journey, a man ran up, knelt down before Him, and asked Him, "Good Teacher, what must I do to inherit eternal life?"*

[18] *"Why do you call Me good?" Jesus asked him. "No one is good but One—God.* [19] *You know the commandments:*

*Do not murder;
do not commit adultery;
do not steal;
do not bear false witness;
do not defraud;
honor your father and mother."*

[20] *He said to Him, "Teacher, I have kept all these from my youth."*

[21] *Then, looking at him, Jesus loved him and said to him, "You lack one thing: Go, sell all you have and give to the poor, and you will have treasure in heaven. Then come, follow Me."* [22] *But he was stunned at this demand, and he went away grieving, because he had many possessions.*

[23] *Jesus looked around and said to His disciples, "How hard it is for those who have wealth to enter the kingdom of God!"* [24] *But the disciples were astonished at His words. Again Jesus said to them, "Children, how hard it is to enter the kingdom of God!* [25] *It is easier for a camel to go through the eye of a needle than for a rich person to enter the kingdom of God."*

[26] *So they were even more astonished, saying to one another, "Then who can be saved?"*

²⁷ Looking at them, Jesus said, "With men it is impossible, but not with God, because all things are possible with God."

²⁸ Peter began to tell Him, "Look, we have left everything and followed You."

²⁹ "I assure you," Jesus said, "there is no one who has left house, brothers or sisters, mother or father, children, or fields because of Me and the gospel, ³⁰ who will not receive 100 times more, now at this time—houses, brothers and sisters, mothers and children, and fields, with persecutions—and eternal life in the age to come. ³¹ But many who are first will be last, and the last first."

No proper reading of the New Testament would allow anyone to correctly conclude that Jesus is calling upon all of His followers to live an ascetic lifestyle (e.g., Luke 19 or 2 Corinthians 9). Jesus, in love, was using hyperbole to point out money was the young man's god.

You've studied and trained hard. You work hard. You've borrowed heavily. You are trying to pay off loans, raise a family, and enjoy fruits of your labor all at the same time. What risks might present regarding your use of your time, talents, and treasure for God's service?

Having time, talents, or treasure to share with others may also mean taking risks and facing persecutions or hardships. It may require uncomfortable choices. How will you prepare for the challenges of stewarding the resources God has given to you (1 Corinthians 4:1-7)?

In conjunction with this passage, read Mark 8:34-38. What will you do?

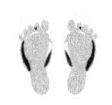

Serving with Humility to Further God's Plan (Mark 10:32-52)

³² They were on the road, going up to Jerusalem, and Jesus was walking ahead of them. They were astonished, but those who followed Him were afraid. Taking the Twelve aside again, He began to tell them the things that would happen to Him.

³³ "Listen! We are going up to Jerusalem. The Son of Man will be handed over to the chief priests and the scribes, and they will condemn Him to death. Then they will hand Him over to the Gentiles, ³⁴ and they will mock Him, spit on Him, flog Him, and kill Him, and He will rise after three days."

³⁵ Then James and John, the sons of Zebedee, approached Him and said, "Teacher, we want You to do something for us if we ask You."

³⁶ "What do you want Me to do for you?" He asked them.

³⁷ They answered Him, "Allow us to sit at Your right and at Your left in Your glory."

³⁸ But Jesus said to them, "You don't know what you're asking. Are you able to drink the cup I drink or to be baptized with the baptism I am baptized with?"

³⁹ "We are able," they told Him.

Jesus said to them, "You will drink the cup I drink, and you will be baptized with the baptism I am baptized with. ⁴⁰ But to sit at My right or left is not Mine to give; instead, it is for those it has been prepared for." ⁴¹ When the other 10 disciples heard this, they began to be indignant with James and John.

⁴² Jesus called them over and said to them, "You know that those who are regarded as rulers of the Gentiles dominate

them, and their men of high positions exercise power over them. ⁴³ *But it must not be like that among you. On the contrary, whoever wants to become great among you must be your servant,* ⁴⁴ *and whoever wants to be first among you must be a slave to all.* ⁴⁵ *For even the Son of Man did not come to be served, but to serve, and to give His life—a ransom for many."*

Jesus was willing to take up His cross. He has called you to take up yours daily. What does taking up your cross mean for you in your practice of healthcare?

In **Romans** 12 the Apostle Paul, intentionally or not, gave a great exposition on Jesus' teaching in Mark 10:35-45.

What strikes you most from these two passages regarding humility as it applies to how you practice healthcare?

Don't Be Blinded by the Limelight
(Mark 10:46-52)

⁴⁶ *They came to Jericho. And as He was leaving Jericho with His disciples and a large crowd, Bartimaeus (the son of Timaeus), a blind beggar, was sitting by the road.* ⁴⁷ *When he heard that it was Jesus the Nazarene, he began to cry out, "Son of David, Jesus, have mercy on me!"* ⁴⁸ *Many people told him to keep quiet, but he was crying out all the more, "Have mercy on me, Son of David!"*

⁴⁹ *Jesus stopped and said, "Call him."*

So they called the blind man and said to him, "Have courage! Get up; He's calling for you." ⁵⁰ *He threw off his coat, jumped up, and came to Jesus.*

⁵¹ *Then Jesus answered him, "What do you want Me to do for you?"*

"Rabbouni," the blind man told Him, "I want to see!"

⁵² *"Go your way," Jesus told him. "Your faith has healed you." Immediately he could see and began to follow Him on the road.*

In light of verses 32-45, how do you see Jesus living out His words in this vignette? To get you started, how did being rich with 'fans' impact the ability of Jesus to hear and respond to the plea of blind Bartimaeus? Contrast that with how the disciples and the crowd apparently failed to see the man's need for a touch from Jesus.

What lesson(s) do you draw for your practice from watching the Master in such a chaotic setting?

Reflection

Major attitudes on display in this study were putting God first, sacrifice, and humility. Yet the excurses was on divorce and adultery. They seem like unrelated themes, but are they?

Describe how having the positive attitudes Jesus commends disciples to have might prevent the negatives that lead to adultery and divorce.

How might you take what you described and use it in teaching patients and peers?

Walking in Jesus' Footsteps Immediately

How are your relationships? Maybe you are married, or you have close friends. You study with classmates and work with a host of coworkers.

Inevitably, relationships get strained, sometimes to the breaking point. Maybe that's happening to you now.

Pray about a strained relationship you might be having. Be vulnerable and honest with God. Is the relationship under stress because you have taken God off the throne of your life, you are not being sacrificial, or your humility just isn't what it needs to be?

Write down the relationship you want to see improve. Then write down which attitude(s) of yours needs improvement help from God's Word and the Holy Spirit. Record the results of letting God help your relationship by renewing *your* mind and transforming *your* life.

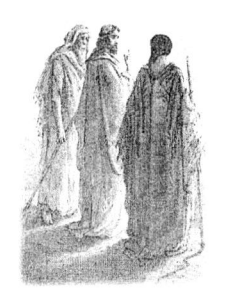

Mark 11

◇

The Double Helix of Public & Self-Deception

Mapping the Path Forward

Mark 11 recounts the beginning of the end of Jesus' healing and teaching ministry in the countryside. Jesus enters Jerusalem or stays nearby to display His compassion for the poor and the hungry, in both metaphorical and physical ways. At the same time, Jesus pictures God's victory over man-made systems that are deceptive, disobedient, and destructive.

Mark uses a pattern of intertwined, alternating accounts of public and self-deception, suggestive of a DNA molecule's double helix construction. Observe how Mark allows you to look at the behavior of others but then drives you to look within yourself lest you think too highly of yourself.

This study continues challenging Christians in healthcare to take a close look at who they are in Christ and what their priorities are. It asks, "Are you willing to deceive yourself and others in order to maintain your sense of control?"

What does this chapter say to Christians in healthcare?

- The heart of Mark 11 is God's desire that the poor and the hungry, the downtrodden and weak be cared for. Power to do that is rooted in faith and faithfulness.

- Faith precedes faithfulness. Faith without deeds is dead, just as deeds not rooted in faith are as filthy rags. Does your faith inform how you practice and does your practice in turn display your faith?

- If the Lord is willing to curse a fig tree that cannot help itself in order to make an object lesson for mankind, how much more will He judge those who have the information necessary to obey Him and bear fruit, yet choose not to do so?

Setting the Stage
(Mark 11:1b)

"at Bethphage and Bethany near the Mount of Olives,"

Bethphage means 'House of Figs.'

Bethany appears to mean 'House of Alms,' or 'House of the Poor.'

The Mount of Olives has numerous olive presses. The olives grown nearby on the hillsides are crushed under massive stones to press out the light, life, and health-giving oil. The Mount of Olives is also where the Garden of Gethsemane is located … the place where Jesus was crushed in tribulation and prayer, to sweat the blood that gives His followers light, life, and healing.

As you might have guessed by now, the use of physical objects or events to teach spiritual lessons – signs – are going to be featured in this chapter. Keep your spiritual vision focused as you answer the questions in this study.

"Triumphal" Entry
(Mark 11:1-11)

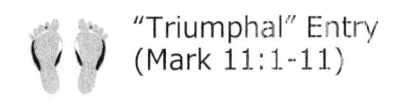

11 ¹*When they approached Jerusalem, at Bethphage and Bethany near the Mount of Olives, He sent two of His disciples* ²*and told them, "Go into the village ahead of you. As soon as you enter it, you will find a young donkey tied there, on which no one has ever sat. Untie it and bring it here.* ³*If anyone says to you, 'Why are you doing this?' say, 'The Lord needs it and will send it back here right away.'"*

⁴*So they went and found a young donkey outside in the street, tied by a door. They untied it,* ⁵*and some of those standing there said to them, "What are you doing, untying the donkey?"* ⁶*They answered them just as Jesus had said, so they let them go.* ⁷*Then they brought the donkey to Jesus and threw their robes on it, and He sat on it.*

⁸*Many people spread their robes on the road, and others spread leafy branches cut from the fields.* ⁹*Then those who went ahead and those who followed kept shouting:*

Hosanna!
He who comes in the name
of the Lord is the blessed One!
¹⁰*The coming kingdom*
of our father David is blessed!
Hosanna in the highest heaven!

¹¹*And He went into Jerusalem and into the temple complex. After looking around at everything, since it was already late, He went out to Bethany with the Twelve.*

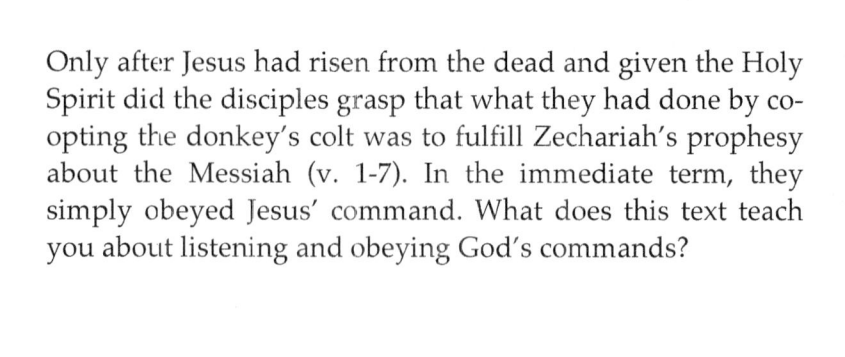

Only after Jesus had risen from the dead and given the Holy Spirit did the disciples grasp that what they had done by co-opting the donkey's colt was to fulfill Zechariah's prophesy about the Messiah (v. 1-7). In the immediate term, they simply obeyed Jesus' command. What does this text teach you about listening and obeying God's commands?

Given the location, what are the likely kinds of branches being spread before Jesus?

From **Genesis 3:7**, what do you think Adam and Eve's use of fig leaves to cover themselves represented?

What do you think Jesus' ride over fig leaves represents?

Verse 11 reminds all of us to be patient. Timing matters. God knows the right time for everything.

The Danger of Fruitlessness
(Mark 11:12-14)

¹² *The next day when they came out from Bethany, He was hungry.* ¹³ *After seeing in the distance a fig tree with leaves, He went to find out if there was anything on it. When He came to it, He found nothing but leaves, because it was not the season for figs.* ¹⁴ *He said to it, "May no one ever eat fruit from you again!" And His disciples heard it.*

All of creation serves God and exists for the benefit of humanity. Jesus was fully human and could experience hunger, especially after spending the night in a poor city. So Jesus begins to build a teaching picture for the disciples by using a fig tree (representing man's schemes regarding salvation) to illustrate the ultimate end for those people who don't produce fruit ... in season and out of season (2 Timothy 4:2).

Man's Interests vs. God's Interests
(Mark 11:15-19)

¹⁵ They came to Jerusalem, and He went into the temple complex and began to throw out those buying and selling in the temple. He overturned the money changers' tables and the chairs of those selling doves, ¹⁶ and would not permit anyone to carry goods through the temple complex.

¹⁷ Then He began to teach them: "Is it not written, My house will be called a house of prayer for all nations. But you have made it a den of thieves!" ¹⁸ Then the chief priests and the scribes heard it and started looking for a way to destroy Him. For they were afraid of Him, because the whole crowd was astonished by His teaching.

¹⁹ And whenever evening came, they would go out of the city.

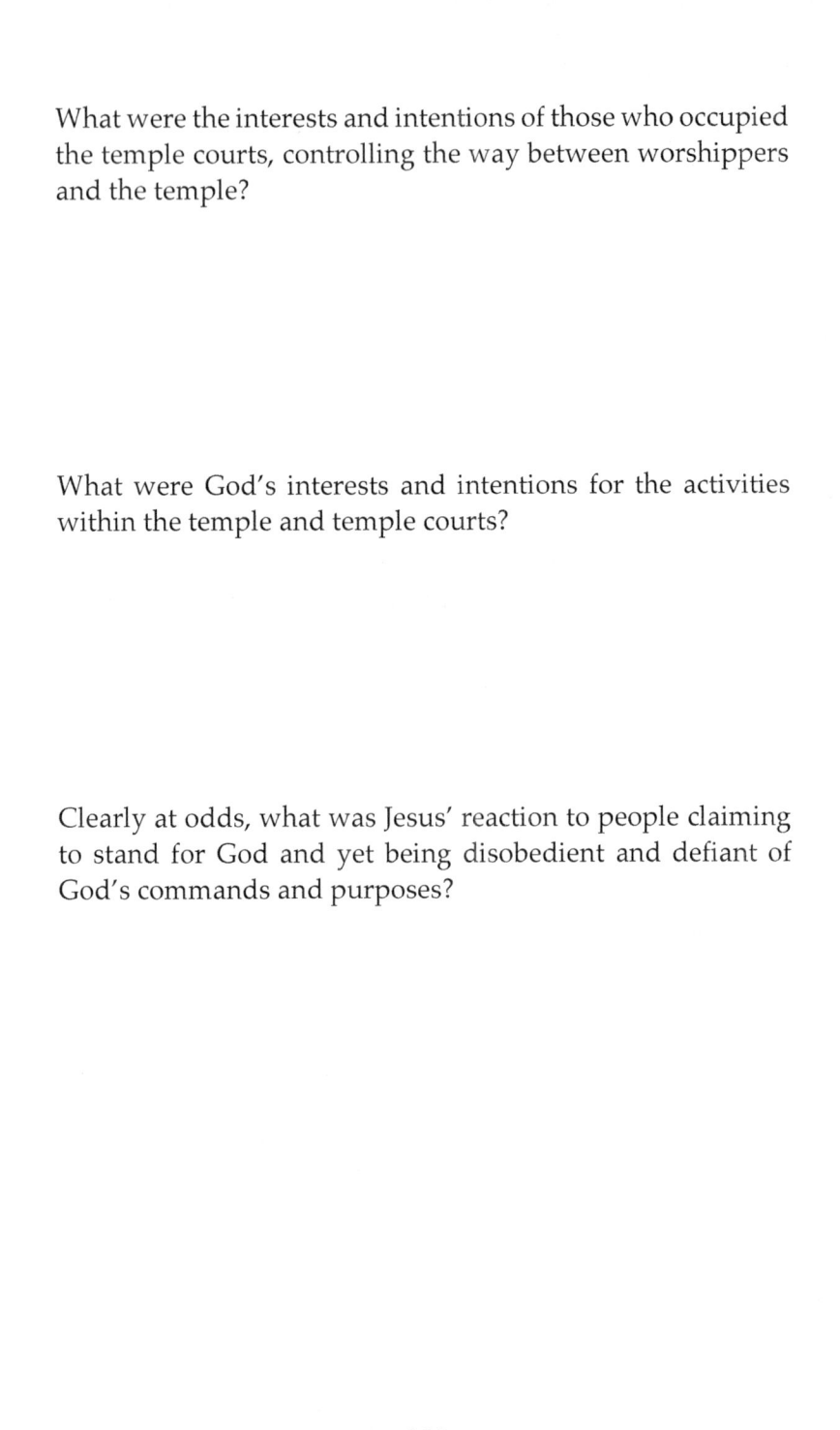

What were the interests and intentions of those who occupied the temple courts, controlling the way between worshippers and the temple?

What were God's interests and intentions for the activities within the temple and temple courts?

Clearly at odds, what was Jesus' reaction to people claiming to stand for God and yet being disobedient and defiant of God's commands and purposes?

Prayer Must Root in Faith, Not Self-Deception (Mark 11:20-26)

[20] *Early in the morning, as they were passing by, they saw the fig tree withered from the roots up.* [21] *Then Peter remembered and said to Him, "Rabbi, look! The fig tree that You cursed is withered."*

[22] *Jesus replied to them, "Have faith in God.* [23] *I assure you: If anyone says to this mountain, 'Be lifted up and thrown into the sea,' and does not doubt in his heart, but believes that what he says will happen, it will be done for him.* [24] *Therefore I tell you, all the things you pray and ask for — believe that you have received them, and you will have them.* [25] *And whenever you stand praying, if you have anything against anyone, forgive him, so that your Father in heaven will also forgive you your wrongdoing. [*[26] *But if you don't forgive, neither will your Father in heaven forgive your wrongdoing.]"*

What did the withered fig tree represent?

What did Jesus say about operating from a position of faith?

Certainly it has crossed your mind that you've never seen a mountain fly. Does that mean Jesus was being hyperbolic about the power of prayer? No. He made the statement within the fuller context of God's view of prayer. Read Deuteronomy 6:16-19, Luke 4:9-12 and 1 John 5:14-15, and Luke 22:39-47a.

What did Jesus say about forgiveness as it relates to prayer? What link do you see between deceiving yourself about your holiness and the effectiveness of your prayers?

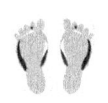

Lost Fellowship with Jesus for the Unrepentant (Mark 11:27-33)

²⁷ *They came again to Jerusalem. As He was walking in the temple complex, the chief priests, the scribes, and the elders came* ²⁸ *and asked Him, "By what authority are You doing these things? Who gave You this authority to do these things?"*

²⁹ *Jesus said to them, "I will ask you one question; then answer Me, and I will tell you by what authority I am doing these things.* ³⁰ *Was John's baptism from heaven or from men? Answer Me."*

³¹ *They began to argue among themselves: "If we say, 'From heaven,' He will say, 'Then why didn't you believe him?'* ³² *But if we say, 'From men'"—they were afraid of the crowd, because everyone thought that John was a genuine prophet.* ³³ *So they answered Jesus, "We don't know."*

And Jesus said to them, "Neither will I tell you by what authority I do these things."

Were the temple leaders tender or hard-hearted toward the things of God?

Using the fig tree metaphor, what is the expected outcome for those too hard-hearted to repent, refusing to produce fruit by faith?

One more thing about figs and sin. Adam fashioned fig leaves into loin cloths for Eve and himself. He was trying to find a way to cover up his guilt and shame. He wanted to hide evidence of their sin, as if God didn't already know about it.

If you were to go outside right now and cut a leaf off a fig tree, over the course of a few days to weeks, what do you think would happen to the fig leaf?

What does that tell you about trying to cover your own sin, rather than confessing it and allowing God to cover you?

Reflection

One of the dangers of practicing healthcare as a vocation is that many people will think highly of you based on your education and experience. If you read too many of your own press clippings, you'll start believing you're something special on your own, apart from God.

What temptations to hubris have come your way through the praises of others?

What safeguards are in place to guard against pride?

Now to real meddling. What sin(s) has God identified in your life that you refuse to lay aside? Why are you being stiff-necked?

Walking in Jesus' Footsteps Immediately

Read **Proverbs 27** carefully, looking for the many references to what it means to be and have a true friend.

Do you have a peer or coworker who is a fellow believer and friend? Do you trust him to speak the truth in love with gentleness and respect?

Ask your friend if he will tell you truthfully where he thinks you might be deceived in some aspect of your personal life or the way you practice healthcare. Note what he says. Be sure to thank him for having the courage to answer your question.

Record a plan for addressing what your friend identified.

Mark 12

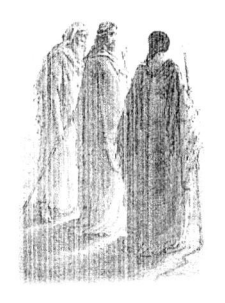

Small Stories
Make for Big Lessons

Mapping the Path Forward

Mark 12 superficially seems like an amalgam of loose ends and tidbits that have nothing at all to do with healthcare. However, embedded in all of these short stories, none of which feature a healing of any sort, are deep and important principles applicable to your healthcare ministry.

This chapter has a great deal to teach Christians in healthcare.

- There is danger in losing sight of who has given you every-thing you have, as well as the responsibility to steward it wisely.

- Often the longest distance to travel is the distance from your head, through your heart, to your hands. It is a distance to be traversed daily in your practice, revealing God's image and likeness.

- If the Apostle Peter needed to be reminded to be faithful in his ministry to feed the sheep, the lambs of God, then it is likely you, too, need to be reminded to be faithful in your Christian healthcare ministry, done in God's name.

Whose Vineyard Is This Anyway?
(Mark 12:1-12)

12 ¹*Then He began to speak to them in parables: "A man planted a vineyard, put a fence around it, dug out a pit for a winepress, and built a watchtower. Then he leased it to tenant farmers and went away. ² At harvest time he sent a slave to the farmers to collect some of the fruit of the vineyard from the farmers. ³ But they took him, beat him, and sent him away empty-handed. ⁴ Again he sent another slave to them, and they hit him on the head and treated him shamefully. ⁵ Then he sent another, and they killed that one. He also sent many others; they beat some and they killed some.*

⁶ *"He still had one to send, a beloved son. Finally he sent him to them, saying, 'They will respect my son.'*

⁷ *"But those tenant farmers said among themselves, 'This is the heir. Come, let's kill him, and the inheritance will be ours!' ⁸ So they seized him, killed him, and threw him out of the vineyard.*

⁹ *"Therefore, what will the owner of the vineyard do? He will come and destroy the farmers and give the vineyard to others. ¹⁰ Haven't you read this Scripture:*

The stone that the builders rejected
has become the cornerstone.
¹¹ This came from the Lord
and is wonderful in our eyes?"

¹² *Because they knew He had said this parable against them, they were looking for a way to arrest Him, but they were afraid of the crowd. So they left Him and went away.*

Who is the vineyard owner?

Read **1 Corinthians 4:6-7, Luke 12:16-21,** and **Deuteronomy 8:11-20**. For you who have studied so diligently and worked so hard, what are the dangers you face as your career and practice grow and generate increasing income, garner you prestige, or isolate you from fellowship and devotional time due to your schedule demands?

What safeguards could you put in place to guard against the dangers you've identified?

Prioritize Properly
(Mark 12:13-17)

[13] Then they sent some of the Pharisees and the Herodians to Him to trap Him by what He said. [14] When they came, they said to Him, "Teacher, we know You are truthful and defer to no one, for You don't show partiality but teach truthfully the way of God. Is it lawful to pay taxes to Caesar or not? [15] Should we pay, or should we not pay?"

But knowing their hypocrisy, He said to them, "Why are you testing Me? Bring Me a denarius to look at." [16] So they brought one. "Whose image and inscription is this?" He asked them.

"Caesar's," they said.

[17] Then Jesus told them, "Give back to Caesar the things that are Caesar's, and to God the things that are God's." And they were amazed at Him.

The coins used for temple offerings had to be of a kind approved by the priests. Unclean Gentile coins had to be traded in for Jewish coins. That's why there was a 'need' for moneychangers in the temple (extracting an exchange-rate profit, of course). That a Pharisee had a Roman denarius coin is his pocket is ironic.

A denarius was considered a day's wage for a common laborer. On the obverse side of some denarius coins of Jesus' day was stamped an image of the emperor Tiberius. The inscription on the reverse side of the coin read, "Caesar Augustus Tiberius, son of the Divine Augustus." Knowing His penchant for using objects as signs, if Jesus was holding up that coin before the crowd, He may have shown the crowd the obverse side of the coin while saying, *"Give back to Caesar the things that are Caesar's."* Then He flipped the coin around to show the crowd the reverse side saying, *"and to God the things that are God's."*

What did the reverse of such a coin claim about Divine Augustus and, by extension, Caesar Augustus Tiberius? (Augustus means 'sacred' or 'revered.' Caesar came to mean 'emperor.')

Therefore, Jesus told the crowd it was possible and right to:

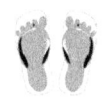

Don't Abandon Bible Study & Application (Mark 12:18-27)

¹⁸ Some Sadducees, who say there is no resurrection, came to Him and questioned Him: ¹⁹ "Teacher, Moses wrote for us that if a man's brother dies, leaves his wife behind, and leaves no child, his brother should take the wife and produce offspring for his brother. ²⁰ There were seven brothers. The first took a wife, and dying, left no offspring. ²¹ The second also took her, and he died, leaving no offspring. And the third likewise. ²² So the seven left no offspring. Last of all, the woman died too. ²³ In the resurrection, when they rise, whose wife will she be, since the seven had married her?"

²⁴ Jesus told them, "Are you not deceived because you don't know the Scriptures or the power of God? ²⁵ For when they rise from the dead, they neither marry nor are given in marriage but are like angels in heaven. ²⁶ Now concerning the dead being raised—haven't you read in the book of Moses, in the passage about the burning bush, how God spoke to him: I am the God of Abraham and the God of Isaac and the God of Jacob? ²⁷ He is not God of the dead but of the living. You are badly deceived."

One danger of being so used to studying and following procedures and protocols, standards of care, and best practices is things become habit, routine, dare we say, boring. If that happens to your medical practice, you may grow to see God as small and distant too – a disengaged artifact of the past. You stop spending time with Him. Eventually your spiritual vision fades, your spiritual hearing dulls, and your spiritual voice waivers.

One negative impact of such a situation is that you become an ineffective ambassador of reconciliation, possibly even making erroneous statements on God's behalf. Left unaddressed, even worse potential impacts of neglecting to spend time with God are that you become a prodigal in a far country or your faith is shipwrecked.

How can fellowship with the saints, prayer, and Bible study help guard you against neglecting or misspeaking for God? For ideas read Hebrews 10:24-25, 1 Thessalonians 5:16-18, and 2 Timothy 3:16-17.

Revealing God's Image and Likeness (Mark 12:28-34)

²⁸ *One of the scribes approached. When he heard them debating and saw that Jesus answered them well, he asked Him, "Which command is the most important of all?"*

²⁹ *"This is the most important," Jesus answered:*

Listen, Israel! The Lord our God, the Lord is One. ³⁰ *Love the Lord your God with all your heart, with all your soul, with all your mind, and with all your strength.*

³¹ *"The second is: Love your neighbor as yourself. There is no other command greater than these."*

³² *Then the scribe said to Him, "You are right, Teacher! You have correctly said that He is One, and there is no one else except Him.* ³³ *And to love Him with all your heart, with all your understanding, and with all your strength, and to love your neighbor as yourself, is far more important than all the burnt offerings and sacrifices."*

³⁴ *When Jesus saw that he answered intelligently, He said to him, "You are not far from the kingdom of God." And no one dared to question Him any longer.*

Jesus says in this passage that the kingdom of God is near you when your head and heart know what to do to please God. That's because you are growing in God's image as He intended. Reading Luke 10:25-37, Romans 12, 1 Peter 2:11-17, 1 John 3:16-24, or James 1:19-25, you discover God's kingdom appears to the world as you display His likeness by doing the good things He intended for you to do.

If you read through these passages, what do they say about what your head and heart think about God having to work through your hands?

Give an example or two of how Bible study, prayer, and Christian fellowship changed the way you think about God, feel about God, and express His likeness through your healthcare practice.

The Holy Spirit and Your Spiritual Voice (Mark 12:35-37)

³⁵ So Jesus asked this question as He taught in the temple complex, "How can the scribes say that the Messiah is the Son of David? ³⁶ David himself says by the Holy Spirit:

The Lord declared to my Lord,
'Sit at My right hand
until I put Your enemies under Your feet.'

³⁷ David himself calls Him 'Lord'; how then can the Messiah be his Son?" And the large crowd was listening to Him with delight.

While you don't speak new revelations as David did, the Holy Spirit still wants to inspire you to speak to those around you with a spiritual voice. Read **John 14:25-26, Acts 1:8,** and **Luke 21:13-15.**

What does the Bible say to you about the Holy Spirit giving you a spiritual voice?

What do these passages tell you are at least some of the reasons you are given a spiritual voice?

Abuse of Power & Position Is Punished Harshly (Mark 12:38-40)

^{38} He also said in His teaching, "Beware of the scribes, who want to go around in long robes, and who want greetings in the marketplaces, ^{39} the front seats in the synagogues, and the places of honor at banquets. ^{40} They devour widows' houses and say long prayers just for show. These will receive harsher punishment."

God is looking to see how faithful you are in the little things before He gives you bigger things to oversee. You already have an important position and power over people through healthcare. You have been afforded great trust by your peers and patients.

What do you think God wants you to be doing with the position, power, and trust you already have?

What will God do to those abusing position, power, or trust?

God Looks at Sacrifice, Not Savings Accounts
(Mark 12:41-44)

⁴¹ *Sitting across from the temple treasury, He watched how the crowd dropped money into the treasury. Many rich people were putting in large sums.* ⁴² *And a poor widow came and dropped in two tiny coins worth very little.* ⁴³ *Summoning His disciples, He said to them, "I assure you: This poor widow has put in more than all those giving to the temple treasury.* ⁴⁴ *For they all gave out of their surplus, but she out of her poverty has put in everything she possessed—all she had to live on."*

Was Jesus commending poverty? Explain your answer.

If you believe Jesus was not advocating destitution, what was He approving in this story?

How do you think this passage applies to what you do with the blessings God gives you?

Reflection

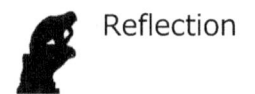

Which of these seven passages resonated the most with you? Why?

List specific ways thinking about these seven passages will affect the way you will provide Christian healthcare to your patients. In other words, how will what you put into your heart and mind come out through your hands?

Walking in Jesus' Footsteps Immediately

Authorities are a gift to humanity, ideally serving for your benefit by promoting good and restraining evil. You are commanded to pray for authorities so that your life may be lived peaceably.

In the account using the denarius coin, you learned that sometimes those in authority overstep their proper bounds. Little 'g' government, for example, thinks of itself as big 'G' God. Or maybe those under authority would prefer to bow down to 'g' as their 'G.'

When authorities go astray, it may be the decision of an individual, or the individual is acting under pressure from external influences. Either way, often there comes an assault on expressing your opinion in the public square. Your right – your Christian obligation – to practice healthcare according to best practices and your conscience as informed by biblical principles is ridiculed, oppressed, financially punished, or even criminalized.

Do you fear or feel an authority acting against your practice?

What is your prayerfully-made plan to deal with your potential fear or current situation?

Mark 13

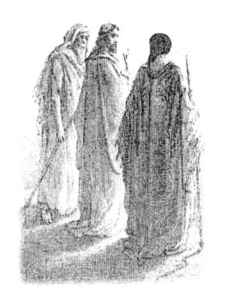

Labor Pain Principles

Mapping the Path Forward

Mark 13 features Jesus teaching His disciples about the end times. In Jesus' prophesies there was the near-term validation, and the yet-to-be fulfilled future. (For example, in the first passage you will examine, Tiberius tearing down the Jerusalem temple in 70 A.D. was a near-term taste of bigger things yet to come.)

The overarching theme of this chapter of Mark is that there will be pressure, persecution, and tribulation for Christ-followers. In this world you will have trouble, and that will extend into your training and your practice too. While this chapter talks about the Great Tribulation as the worst trouble of all, you will find this study picks up on Jesus' labor pain motif to teach about handling challenges common to all Christians.

What will this chapter have to say to Christians in healthcare?

- All people face pressure. Christians will face additional stresses because of their faith.

- It is sometimes okay to leave the place of pressure.

- It is not okay to leave Jesus to get the pressure to stop.

- Enduring, persevering, and overcoming all result in special blessings.

What Will Endure?
(Mark 13:1-2)

13 ¹*As He was going out of the temple complex, one of His disciples said to Him, "Teacher, look! What massive stones! What impressive buildings!"*

²*Jesus said to him, "Do you see these great buildings? Not one stone will be left here on another that will not be thrown down!"*

What was the disciple impressed by?

Nothing has changed. In "Thrown Down," (Notes of Encouragement, Durham, Christian Healthcare Insights, 2016, pp. 60-61), I wrote about modern healthcare,

> "Huge, very imposing complexes are filled with medical priests and priestesses and their gargantuan support staffs. One used to look at the staff of Asclepius as the symbol of medicine. Today, one might argue, the healthcare symbol is the 10-15 story high cantilever crane."

Read **Hebrews 12:25-29** and **2 Peter 3:1-13**. What is the future for all man-made structures and systems?

How much eternal value is in these structures and systems?

The Principle of Labor Pains
(Mark 13:3-8)

³ *While He was sitting on the Mount of Olives across from the temple complex, Peter, James, John, and Andrew asked Him privately,* ⁴ *"Tell us, when will these things happen? And what will be the sign when all these things are about to take place?"*

⁵ *Then Jesus began by telling them: "Watch out that no one deceives you.* ⁶ *Many will come in My name, saying, 'I am He,' and they will deceive many.* ⁷ *When you hear of wars and rumors of wars, don't be alarmed; these things must take place, but the end is not yet.* ⁸ *For nation will rise up against nation, and kingdom against kingdom. There will be earthquakes in various places, and famines. These are the beginning of birth pains.*

The image of labor pains is a common motif in Scripture. It was a favorite metaphor used by Jesus. Take note of why.

Labor has increased pain because of si___ (See Genesis 3:6, 16a).

With modern medicine, contractions can be slowed or stopped temporarily. However, especially at the time Jesus used the metaphor, under normal and natural circumstances contractions cannot be st_____.

During labor, waves of contractions increase in fr_____ and am_____.

The contractions of painful labor are intended to ultimately result in the bi_____ of something new and beautiful.

How does this labor pain imagery prepare you to deal with troubles in your practice?

Labor Endured, Joy Delivered
(Mark 13:9-13)

⁹ *"But you, be on your guard! They will hand you over to sanhedrins, and you will be flogged in the synagogues. You will stand before governors and kings because of Me, as a witness to them.* ¹⁰ *And the good news must first be proclaimed to all nations.* ¹¹ *So when they arrest you and hand you over, don't worry beforehand what you will say. On the contrary, whatever is given to you in that hour—say it. For it isn't you speaking, but the Holy Spirit.* ¹² *Then brother will betray brother to death, and a father his child. Children will rise up against parents and put them to death.* ¹³ *And you will be hated by everyone because of My name. But the one who endures to the end will be delivered.*

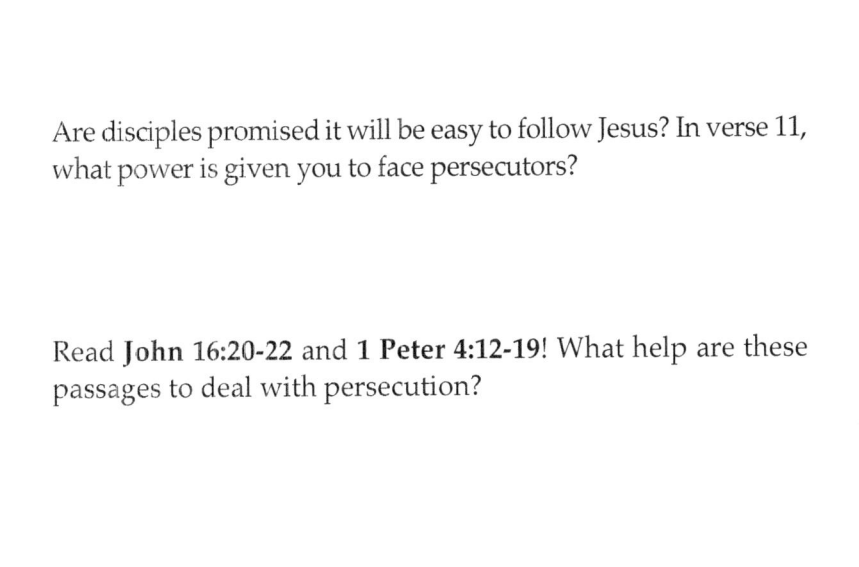

Are disciples promised it will be easy to follow Jesus? In verse 11, what power is given you to face persecutors?

Read **John 16:20-22** and **1 Peter 4:12-19**! What help are these passages to deal with persecution?

Along with many of King David's psalms, these passages reveal the importance of trusting God despite persecutions. Jot down your thoughts after each one you choose to read:

- Matthew 10:21-22, 24:12-13

- 1 Corinthians 4:11-16, 13:6-7

- 2 Timothy 2:12-13, 3:10-11, 4:5

- Hebrews 12:2-7

- James 1:12

- 1 Peter 2:19-20

Sometimes It Is Okay to Flee
(Mark 13:14-23)

¹⁴ *"When you see the abomination that causes desolation standing where it should not" (let the reader understand), "then those in Judea must flee to the mountains!* ¹⁵ *A man on the housetop must not come down or go in to get anything out of his house.* ¹⁶ *And a man in the field must not go back to get his clothes.* ¹⁷ *Woe to pregnant women and nursing mothers in those days!* ¹⁸ *Pray it won't happen in winter.* ¹⁹ *For those will be days of tribulation, the kind that hasn't been from the beginning of the world, which God created, until now and never will be again!* ²⁰ *Unless the Lord limited those days, no one would survive. But He limited those days because of the elect, whom He chose.*

²¹ *"Then if anyone tells you, 'Look, here is the Messiah! Look—there!' do not believe it!* ²² *For false messiahs and false prophets will rise up and will perform signs and wonders to lead astray, if possible, the elect.* ²³ *And you must watch! I have told you everything in advance.*

Jesus permitted disciples to leave unwelcoming places.

Paul fled places when severe persecution broke out against him.

When dross has been fully burned off, there is no reason to leave gold in the fire.

There are times it is okay to leave a high pressure situation, but be sure it is the right time and for the right reason. Forcing all labor pains to stop may ultimately lead to a stillbirth. Don't short circuit God's work to purify and prove you, and shortchange your blessing.

What are some 'false messiahs' that might lead you to leave a hard situation prematurely?

What tools do you have to help determine that leaving a difficult situation is what God would have you do?

The Doctor Is Coming
(Mark 13:24-27)

^{24} *"But in those days, after that tribulation:*

The sun will be darkened,
and the moon will not shed its light;
^{25} the stars will be falling from the sky,
and the celestial powers will be shaken.

^{26} Then they will see the Son of Man coming in clouds with great power and glory. ^{27} He will send out the angels and gather His elect from the four winds, from the end of the earth to the end of the sky.

Even though your labor is painful, it is not permanent. The Great Physician is on the way to your delivery room. You will see the face of Jesus, though it may not be as soon as you would like.

Describe a situation where it felt like the stars were falling from the sky onto your head, and the ground under your feet was but quaking sand.

If you didn't know Jesus at the time, how did you handle the trial? If you did, did you seek His help? How did He help?

Lean on God's Word, Not a Grapevine (Mark 13:28-31)

[28] *"Learn this parable from the fig tree: As soon as its branch becomes tender and sprouts leaves, you know that summer is near.* [29] *In the same way, when you see these things happening, know that He is near—at the door!* [30] *I assure you: This generation will certainly not pass away until all these things take place.* [31] *Heaven and earth will pass away, but My words will never pass away.*

God is the author of feelings and emotions. Therefore, according to His Word, they are very good. They can produce fruit. However, when the pressure is on, feelings have a way of becoming the staff on which you lean.

Read **Ezekiel 15:1-5**.

If you try to hang something heavy on a grapevine peg, contra a peg made of tree wood, what will happen to the heavy object?

Even if it appears to be fruitful, of what *enduring* value is a grapevine?

According to Mark 13:31, what is ever-enduring – worthy to put your whole weight on when labor pains are too much to bear?

Read John 1:14 and Matthew 11:28-30. What are your thoughts about letting God help you bear up during labor pains?

Be Alert!
(Mark 13:32-37)

³² "Now concerning that day or hour no one knows—neither the angels in heaven nor the Son—except the Father. ³³ Watch! Be alert! For you don't know when the time is coming. ³⁴ It is like a man on a journey, who left his house, gave authority to his slaves, gave each one his work, and commanded the doorkeeper to be alert. ³⁵ Therefore be alert, since you don't know when the master of the house is coming—whether in the evening or at midnight or at the crowing of the rooster or early in the morning. ³⁶ Otherwise, he might come suddenly and find you sleeping. ³⁷ And what I say to you, I say to everyone: Be alert!"

People have gotten pretty good at estimating a baby's due date. Often the mother or the couple will assemble a 'jump kit' to take to the hospital with them when the labor pains begin. Yet the due date remains only an educated guess, based upon various factors and signs. When the labor pains begin, they always seem to surprise those involved. The biggest surprise, and potentially most complicated, is when the labor begins before preparations have been made.

Don't let the labor pains or the pleasures of your profession make you dull to your spiritual situation. You've been born again. Jesus has a claim on your life, and will use trials to discipline, shape, and mature you for His service. In all circumstances, you remain His ambassador and laborer in the field. As you continue to provide excellent care, remain alert to the Master who called you to it.

Reflection

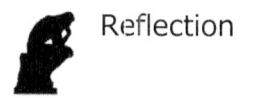

This study of Mark 13 contained suggestions and assignments to read 17 ancillary passages – far more than any other study in this book. The reason for recommending them was because healthcare, as a calling and a profession, is undergoing dramatic and arguably highly unhealthy change.

Much of the change is driven by change in the culture in which your care is set. If you dispassionately step back and look at the big picture, you may notice striking similarities between the cultures of pre-Constantine Rome and today, including conflicting views on the value of all life, at all stages, and in all states of ability. In the Roman empire, saints were often persecuted for living a faith informed by God's Word. Such trials are now happening in your culture.

Of all the ancillary passages you read, describe which ones spoke to your spirit and how the passages have given you encouragement, strength, or wisdom to endure.

Walking in Jesus' Footsteps Immediately

Contact information for your State Senator:

Contact information for your State Representative:

Contact Information for your U.S. Senators:

Contact information for your U.S. Representative:

Contact each one. Tell them you are praying for them, presumably because God says to. Offer to be available to them to answer questions that they may have regarding healthcare. Be an agent of God's grace and wisdom.

Mark 14

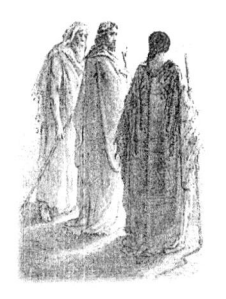

◇

Will You Be Found Faithful?

Mapping the Path Forward

Mark 14 highlights the events surrounding Jesus' surrender of Himself into the hands of men. Clearly He and His work are the most critical aspects of the chapter. Yet this chapter also has much to teach you about your faithfulness to your eternal calling to God and to those you serve through your healthcare ministry.

This study says to Christians in healthcare:

- You may have a willing spirit, but your flesh is weak.

- You can't fulfill your mission apart from prayerfully seeking God's power.

- You fool yourself if you think you are above failing as a minister and ambassador for God through healthcare.

- Jesus knows your weaknesses. He may admonish, but He never condemns you for it.

Power and Conspiracy Against God
(Mark 14:1-2)

14 *¹After two days it was the Passover and the Festival of Unleavened Bread. The chief priests and the scribes were looking for a treacherous way to arrest and kill Him. ² "Not during the festival," they said, "or there may be rioting among the people."*

Read **Psalm 2:1-6**.

In the psalm, all people are guilty of plotting against God. The ones in power, who have authority, are singled out for scheming against God so as not to be under His authority. Whether in Psalm 2:1-6 or here in Mark 2:1-2, notice that the treachery and conspiracy among people with power or authority isn't one person against God. Rather, it is a collective attack. They egg each other on approvingly.

Can God's plans be overthrown or He be dethroned by men?

Who are those in authority within your circle of associates who tempt others – maybe even yourself – to undermine or overthrow God or other people?

How can you avoid being drawn into treacherous schemes?

The Nobility & Ignobility of Humanity
(Mark 14:3-11)

³ *While He was in Bethany at the house of Simon who had a serious skin disease, as He was reclining at the table, a woman came with an alabaster jar of pure and expensive fragrant oil of nard. She broke the jar and poured it on His head.* ⁴ *But some were expressing indignation to one another: "Why has this fragrant oil been wasted?* ⁵ *For this oil might have been sold for more than 300 denarii and given to the poor." And they began to scold her.*

⁶ *Then Jesus said, "Leave her alone. Why are you bothering her? She has done a noble thing for Me.* ⁷ *You always have the poor with you, and you can do what is good for them whenever you want, but you do not always have Me.* ⁸ *She has done what she could; she has anointed My body in advance for burial.* ⁹ *I assure you: Wherever the gospel is proclaimed in the whole world, what this woman has done will also be told in memory of her."*

¹⁰ *Then Judas Iscariot, one of the Twelve, went to the chief priests to hand Him over to them.* ¹¹ *And when they heard this, they were glad and promised to give him silver. So he started looking for a good opportunity to betray Him.*

You probably chose healthcare as a vocation for n_____ reasons. You wanted to serve people.

Yet, when despair over slow or no progress, frustrations, economic pressures, and/or greed for reputation or power enter into your calculations, have you found yourself becoming indignant and acting ignobly?

God calls upon His people to avoid sin at such times by giving Him responsibility for redeeming situations which tempt you to become indignant or act ignobly.

Humble yourselves, therefore, under the mighty hand of God, so that He may exalt you at the proper time.

1 Peter 5:6

Humble yourselves before the Lord, and He will exalt you.

James 4:10

Teammates and Your Referral Network
(Mark 14:12-16)

¹² *On the first day of Unleavened Bread, when they sacrifice the Passover lamb, His disciples asked Him, "Where do You want us to go and prepare the Passover so You may eat it?"*

¹³ *So He sent two of His disciples and told them, "Go into the city, and a man carrying a water jug will meet you. Follow him.* ¹⁴ *Wherever he enters, tell the owner of the house, 'The Teacher says, "Where is the guest room for Me to eat the Passover with My disciples?"' * ¹⁵ *He will show you a large room upstairs, furnished and ready. Make the preparations for us there."* ¹⁶ *So the disciples went out, entered the city, and found it just as He had told them, and they prepared the Passover.*

CRITICAL QUESTIONS

Read **Acts 18:5-11** and **1 Kings 19:1-18**.

From all three passages, what principle(s) do you draw out about the Lord making provision for His work through you?

What important practical action(s) should this lead you to take in your workplace?

Healthcare practitioners often have to make referrals, either due to time constraints or expertise. Why is it particularly and especially crucial Christians in healthcare develop not only a support network (see the Mark 3:31-35 module), but a referral network of other Christian practitioners and chaplains who are also dedicated to treating the whole patient?

Not Everyone Is On the Lord's Team (Mark 14:17-21)

17 When evening came, He arrived with the Twelve. 18 While they were reclining and eating, Jesus said, "I assure you: One of you will betray Me—one who is eating with Me!"

19 They began to be distressed and to say to Him one by one, "Surely not I?"

20 He said to them, "It is one of the Twelve—the one who is dipping bread with Me in the bowl. 21 For the Son of Man will go just as it is written about Him, but woe to that man by whom the Son of Man is betrayed! It would have been better for that man if he had not been born."

Judas may have started out with good intentions but grew disenchanted with the direction of Jesus' ministry compared to what Judas wanted or expected. Or, Judas put on airs as a disciple and was always in it for himself.

Pressures for power, promotion, publication, and popularity creep into healthcare teams like everywhere else. You don't always get to pick your team, but where possible, don't be unequally yoked to someone who doesn't have a Christian worldview. Where unavoidable, be wise as serpents but gentle as doves.

Even though Jesus always knew Judas would betray Him, (omniscience has its advantages), He still chose him, sent him on ministry assignments, and treated him generally like every other disciple. Only after Judas took steps to betray Jesus did Jesus act.

What lessons do you draw from seeing how Jesus handled Judas as a potential and then actual betrayer?

A Covenant for Many, Now and Future (Mark 14:22-26)

²² *As they were eating, He took bread, blessed and broke it, gave it to them, and said, "Take it; this is My body."*

²³ *Then He took a cup, and after giving thanks, He gave it to them, and so they all drank from it.* ²⁴ *He said to them, "This is My blood that establishes the covenant; it is shed for many.* ²⁵ *I assure you: I will no longer drink of the fruit of the vine until that day when I drink it in a new way in the kingdom of God."* ²⁶ *After singing psalms, they went out to the Mount of Olives.*

What spiritual lesson do you draw from the immediate connection between Jesus sharing the fruit of the vine – a product of the wine press – and His departing to the Mount of Olives? (Hint: See the Mark 11:1b module notes.)

Read **2 Corinthians 5:16-6:2**. Through the breaking of His body and the shedding of His blood, God has established a new covenant through faith, in order to make available an eternal hope of life with God. However, as Jesus exemplified, eating and drinking without explanatory words is just a meal. That's why you are called to be His ambassadors of reconciliation. Whether in written or spoken word, ambassadors are not to be silent. They are God's chosen agents to give voice to His will and works.

For whom was the body and blood of Jesus given?

As God's ambassador of reconciliation, you should be willing to share that message with whom?

Notice the disciples left singing psalms. Just as God gave insulin so energy-laden glucose can enter a cell, He gave music to humans so His Word can readily and enduringly enter a person's soul. Thus the Apostle Paul's commission in Ephesians 5:19 and Colossians 3:16.

Be Honest in Your Self-Assessment
(Mark 14:27-31)

²⁷ Then Jesus said to them, "All of you will run away, because it is written:

I will strike the shepherd,
and the sheep will be scattered.

²⁸ But after I have been resurrected, I will go ahead of you to Galilee."

²⁹ Peter told Him, "Even if everyone runs away, I will certainly not!"

³⁰ "I assure you," Jesus said to him, "today, this very night, before the rooster crows twice, you will deny Me three times!"

³¹ But he kept insisting, "If I have to die with You, I will never deny You!" And they all said the same thing.

Was Peter the only one sure of himself?

What warning about yourself do you draw from this?

Review Romans 12:3.

Stay with Me, Pray for Yourselves
(Mark 14:32-42)

[32] Then they came to a place named Gethsemane, and He told His disciples, "Sit here while I pray." [33] He took Peter, James, and John with Him, and He began to be deeply distressed and horrified. [34] Then He said to them, "My soul is swallowed up in sorrow —to the point of death. Remain here and stay awake." [35] Then He went a little farther, fell to the ground, and began to pray that if it were possible, the hour might pass from Him. [36] And He said, "Abba, Father! All things are possible for You. Take this cup away from Me. Nevertheless, not what I will, but what You will."

[37] Then He came and found them sleeping. "Simon, are you sleeping?" He asked Peter. "Couldn't you stay awake one hour? [38] Stay awake and pray so that you won't enter into temptation. The spirit is willing, but the flesh is weak."

[39] Once again He went away and prayed, saying the same thing. [40] And He came again and found them sleeping, because they could not keep their eyes open. They did not know what to say to Him. [41] Then He came a third time and said to them, "Are you still sleeping and resting? Enough! The time has come. Look, the Son of Man is being betrayed into the hands of sinners. [42] Get up; let's go! See—My betrayer is near."

Jesus only asked the disciples to keep watch with Him. He initiated and did most of the praying in the Garden of Gethsemane. After all, He was the one in the dire circumstance. (See James 5:13-20 as an application of this.)

Will you be found faithful to keep watch with your patients when they are in dire circumstances?

When the disciples failed to keep watch with and over Jesus, Jesus commanded them to pray they would not fall into temptation. Temptation to what? (Don't say sleep. It is not a sin. However, sleeping was a sign of improper priorities.)

Jesus knew from Zechariah 13:7 that He would be struck and the sheep would scatter. He would be left alone. He wanted to avoid this for as long as possible.

When your patients face dire circumstances and/or death, will you pray with them? Or will you fall asleep in the face of their anguish, in effect abandoning them?

High Pressure and Unexpected Responses (Mark 14:43-52)

⁴³ *While He was still speaking, Judas, one of the Twelve, suddenly arrived. With him was a mob, with swords and clubs, from the chief priests, the scribes, and the elders.* ⁴⁴ *His betrayer had given them a signal. "The One I kiss," he said, "He's the One; arrest Him and take Him away under guard."* ⁴⁵ *So when he came, he went right up to Him and said, "Rabbi!"—and kissed Him.* ⁴⁶ *Then they took hold of Him and arrested Him.* ⁴⁷ *And one of those who stood by drew his sword, struck the high priest's slave, and cut off his ear.*

⁴⁸ *But Jesus said to them, "Have you come out with swords and clubs, as though I were a criminal, to capture Me?* ⁴⁹ *Every day I was among you, teaching in the temple complex, and you didn't arrest Me. But the Scriptures must be fulfilled."* ⁵⁰ *Then they all deserted Him and ran away.*

⁵¹ *Now a certain young man, having a linen cloth wrapped around his naked body, was following Him. They caught hold of him,* ⁵² *but he left the linen cloth behind and ran away naked.*

When the pressure is really bearing down on someone, often the first reaction is to thrash about with a fleshly response, like slashing with a sword.

Describe a time you were tempted to violence by a high pressure situation?

What were the consequences?

Did the violence ultimately help or hurt you?

Many expositors believe Mark was the "certain young man." In theory, he might have left out the highly embarrassing account in verses 51-52, as other Gospel writers did. Yet Mark and the Holy Spirit gave you these facts. What lesson(s) do you draw?

They All Condemned Him
(Mark 14:53-65)

⁵³ *They led Jesus away to the high priest, and all the chief priests, the elders, and the scribes convened.* ⁵⁴ *Peter followed Him at a distance, right into the high priest's courtyard. He was sitting with the temple police, warming himself by the fire.*

⁵⁵ *The chief priests and the whole Sanhedrin were looking for testimony against Jesus to put Him to death, but they could find none.* ⁵⁶ *For many were giving false testimony against Him, but the testimonies did not agree.* ⁵⁷ *Some stood up and were giving false testimony against Him, stating,* ⁵⁸ *"We heard Him say, 'I will demolish this sanctuary made by human hands, and in three days I will build another not made by hands.'"* ⁵⁹ *Yet their testimony did not agree even on this.*

⁶⁰ *Then the high priest stood up before them all and questioned Jesus, "Don't You have an answer to what these men are testifying against You?"* ⁶¹ *But He kept silent and did not answer anything. Again the high priest questioned Him, "Are You the Messiah, the Son of the Blessed One?"*

⁶² *"I am," said Jesus, "and all of you will see the Son of Man seated at the right hand of the Power and coming with the clouds of heaven."*

⁶³ *Then the high priest tore his robes and said, "Why do we still need witnesses?* ⁶⁴ *You have heard the blasphemy! What is your decision?"*

And they all condemned Him to be deserving of death. ⁶⁵ *Then some began to spit on Him, to blindfold Him, and to beat Him, saying, "Prophesy!" The temple police also took Him and slapped Him.*

Verses 53 and 64 use the word "all." That rules out exceptions or excuses. All the religious rulers were present, participated, and agreed on the course of action – killing Jesus.

Remember that mixed into the Sanhedrin were Nicodemus & Joseph of Arimathea who less than 24 hours later would, in a very dangerous atmosphere, reveal themselves to be disciples of Jesus too. And unlike the disciples who had lived with Jesus for three years, Joseph and Nicodemus didn't wait to expose themselves until after the resurrection.

Every follower of Jesus is subject to denying Him at some point and under some form of pressure. What makes the record of Nicodemus and Joseph striking and noteworthy, however, is the speed at which they apparently realized their mistake and made efforts to atone for it.

Have you made a mistake in the way you relate to God or serve Him through your healthcare ministry?

Have you made an attempt to atone for it, including confession to God and repentance?

If not, why? What are you waiting for?

The Scope of Denial Is Complete
(Mark 14:66-72)

⁶⁶ *While Peter was in the courtyard below, one of the high priest's servants came.* ⁶⁷ *When she saw Peter warming himself, she looked at him and said, "You also were with that Nazarene, Jesus."*

⁶⁸ *But he denied it: "I don't know or understand what you're talking about!" Then he went out to the entryway, and a rooster crowed.*

⁶⁹ *When the servant saw him again she began to tell those standing nearby, "This man is one of them!"*

⁷⁰ *But again he denied it. After a little while those standing there said to Peter again, "You certainly are one of them, since you're also a Galilean!"*

⁷¹ *Then he started to curse and to swear with an oath, "I don't know this man you're talking about!"*

⁷² *Immediately a rooster crowed a second time, and Peter remembered when Jesus had spoken the word to him, "Before the rooster crows twice, you will deny Me three times." When he thought about it, he began to weep.*

A careful reading of Matthew's parallel account clearly suggests that Peter, in fear, not only denied Jesus, but also his fellow disciples and his own heritage. Mark abandoned his outer garments in fear. Peter abandoned his inner being.

What do you think Peter was weeping about?

What do you think about the possibility that Peter was weeping out of a fear God would abandon him as completely as Peter had abandoned God, his disciples, and his heritage?

Reflection

Read **3 John**.

How do you see many of the issues raised and principles taught in this study playing out in John's letter?

What activities are commended?

How did John say he would deal with people committing uncommendable actions?

Walking in Jesus' Footsteps Immediately

Reflecting on your ability to fail serves to admonish and teach you. **Failures are not what define you though.** They are not your end, for you are a child of God, assured of an eternal future with Jesus through faith in His person and work.

What hope do you take in how Jesus treated the people around Him when they failed?

Make some notes about how you can communicate God's desire and willingness to redeem to a patient or peer who feels he has done something so bad God doesn't love him, is angry with him, or is using his illness to punish him.

Mark 15

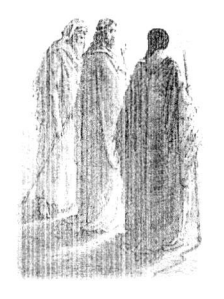

Prepare for Spiritual Warfare

Mapping the Path Forward

Mark 15 is yet another chapter leading you to be very introspective. In the face of severe disrespect and challenges, Jesus models important methods of conduct.

What will this chapter have to say to Christians in healthcare?

- It will not always be easy to be a public follower of Jesus.

- The best answers aren't always words but sometimes your works.

- Despite your best efforts, some situations deteriorate. Are you ready?

- Are you willing to take a risk for Jesus?

Good Works Can Answer On Your Behalf
(Mark 15:1-5)

15 *¹As soon as it was morning, the chief priests had a meeting with the elders, scribes, and the whole Sanhedrin. After tying Jesus up, they led Him away and handed Him over to Pilate.*

² So Pilate asked Him, "Are You the King of the Jews?"

He answered him, "You have said it."

³ And the chief priests began to accuse Him of many things. ⁴ Then Pilate questioned Him again, "Are You not answering anything? Look how many things they are accusing You of!" ⁵ But Jesus still did not answer anything, so Pilate was amazed.

In Jesus' confrontation with Pilate, He answered statements that were true but remained silent regarding false accusations. His reply to the false accusations was in fact the record of the way He conducted His life doing good works. Your good works, to which you were called and which you carry out faithfully and publicly, can go a long way toward being your advocate in times of dispute.

What do the following statements have to say about the works you do as a Christian in healthcare?

- Ephesians 2:10

- Matthew 5:16

- John 10:32

- 1 Timothy 5:25

- Titus 2:7, 14

- Titus 3:8, 14

- 1 Peter 2:12

Not Everyone in Authority Is Brave or Upright (Mark 15:6-15)

⁶ At the festival it was Pilate's custom to release for the people a prisoner they requested. ⁷ There was one named Barabbas, who was in prison with rebels who had committed murder during the rebellion. ⁸ The crowd came up and began to ask Pilate to do for them as was his custom. ⁹ So Pilate answered them, "Do you want me to release the King of the Jews for you?" ¹⁰ For he knew it was because of envy that the chief priests had handed Him over. ¹¹ But the chief priests stirred up the crowd so that he would release Barabbas to them instead.

¹² Pilate asked them again, "Then what do you want me to do with the One you call the King of the Jews?"

¹³ Again they shouted, "Crucify Him!"

¹⁴ Then Pilate said to them, "Why? What has He done wrong?"

But they shouted, "Crucify Him!" all the more.

¹⁵ Then, willing to gratify the crowd, Pilate released Barabbas to them. And after having Jesus flogged, he handed Him over to be crucified.

Name a boss you have had who wouldn't stick up for right.

How did that sort of 'leadership' make you feel?

How did you respond or relate to that person?

Clearly, Jesus was a prisoner by the set purpose of the Father. He would not go free. However, within the context of this study, you are thinking about being an employee, not a prisoner. Imagine you are working for someone who thinks negatively of you and is threatening your job or making it hard for you. Read **Luke 6:27-36** and then **Acts 13:42-52** and **22:22-29**. What are some Christian responses to a hostile employment situation you glean from these passages?

Bullies
(Mark 15:16-20)

¹⁶ *Then the soldiers led Him away into the courtyard (that is, headquarters) and called the whole company together.* ¹⁷ *They dressed Him in a purple robe, twisted together a crown of thorns, and put it on Him.* ¹⁸ *And they began to salute Him, "Hail, King of the Jews!"* ¹⁹ *They kept hitting Him on the head with a reed and spitting on Him. Getting down on their knees, they were paying Him homage.* ²⁰ *When they had mocked Him, they stripped Him of the purple robe, put His clothes on Him, and led Him out to crucify Him.*

Your first reaction to this passage is to think about how you would respond in such a situation. Recognizing how horrible such a situation would be, your second thought might be that you are glad such a thing could never happen to you. Yet, have you thought about going on a medical mission? Missionaries are taken prisoner, abused, tortured, and killed all the time.

Think again. How would you feel in such a situation?

Victims of human trafficking are often treated in such shameful ways. As a Christian, you have a responsibility to step up in defense of those being bullied by traffickers. As a Christian in healthcare, one could argue it is your duty to be informed on how to recognize and help rescue those in such bondage, when they present in your practice.

If you've never studied the issue of human trafficking, or learned how to recognize and help rescue its victims, visit: https://cmda.org/ministry/detail/commission-on-human-trafficking.

Responding to Mocking
(Mark 15:21-32)

²¹ They forced a man coming in from the country, who was passing by, to carry Jesus' cross. He was Simon, a Cyrenian, the father of Alexander and Rufus. ²² And they brought Jesus to the place called Golgotha (which means Skull Place). ²³ They tried to give Him wine mixed with myrrh, but He did not take it. ²⁴ Then they crucified Him and divided His clothes, casting lots for them to decide what each would get. ²⁵ Now it was nine in the morning when they crucified Him. ²⁶ The inscription of the charge written against Him was: THE KING OF THE JEWS.

²⁷ They crucified two criminals with Him, one on His right and one on His left. [²⁸ So the Scripture was fulfilled that says: And He was counted among outlaws.] ²⁹ Those who passed by were yelling insults at Him, shaking their heads, and saying, "Ha! The One who would demolish the sanctuary and build it in three days, ³⁰ save Yourself by coming down from the cross!" ³¹ In the same way, the chief priests with the scribes were mocking Him to one another and saying, "He saved others; He cannot save Himself! ³² Let the Messiah, the King of Israel, come down now from the cross, so that we may see and believe." Even those who were crucified with Him were taunting Him.

Read **Proverbs 9:7-8**.

How should you not respond to mocking of your faith and practice rooted in that faith?

Who should you rebuke, and why?

Read **Matthew 5:43-48** and **Luke 23:34**.

What did Jesus teach and model as the correct response to mockers?

The Observers of Words & Works
(Mark 15:33-41)

³³ When it was noon, darkness came over the whole land until three in the afternoon. ³⁴ And at three Jesus cried out with a loud voice, "Eloi, Eloi, lemá sabachtháni?" which is translated, "My God, My God, why have You forsaken Me?"

³⁵ When some of those standing there heard this, they said, "Look, He's calling for Elijah!" ³⁶ Someone ran and filled a sponge with sour wine, fixed it on a reed, offered Him a drink, and said, "Let's see if Elijah comes to take Him down!"

³⁷ But Jesus let out a loud cry and breathed His last. ³⁸ Then the curtain of the sanctuary was split in two from top to bottom. ³⁹ When the centurion, who was standing opposite Him, saw the way He breathed His last, he said, "This man really was God's Son!"

⁴⁰ There were also women looking on from a distance. Among them were Mary Magdalene, Mary the mother of James the younger and of Joses, and Salome. ⁴¹ When He was in Galilee, they would follow Him and help Him. Many other women had come up with Him to Jerusalem.

As you practice, who might be watching and listening to you? If you need a reminder or hint, review your study of Mark 2.

Describe what the Roman centurion saw and didn't see during Jesus' passion.

How did the centurion respond to what he heard and observed?

What does his example say to you about being consistent in your words and works within your vocational environment?

Step Out of the Shadows
(Mark 15:42-47)

⁴² *When it was already evening, because it was preparation day (that is, the day before the Sabbath),* ⁴³ *Joseph of Arimathea, a prominent member of the Sanhedrin who was himself looking forward to the kingdom of God, came and boldly went in to Pilate and asked for Jesus' body.* ⁴⁴ *Pilate was surprised that He was already dead. Summoning the centurion, he asked him whether He had already died.* ⁴⁵ *When he found out from the centurion, he gave the corpse to Joseph.* ⁴⁶ *After he bought some fine linen, he took Him down and wrapped Him in the linen. Then he placed Him in a tomb cut out of the rock, and rolled a stone against the entrance to the tomb.* ⁴⁷ *Now Mary Magdalene and Mary the mother of Joses were watching where He was placed.*

It is very instructive to read all of the Gospel accounts of Joseph of Arimathea and Nicodemus, Israel's teacher. They were the academics of their day. They clearly were searching for the coming kingdom of God.

At some point they may have thought they had found its king in Jesus. Apparently however, peer pressure from the other academics caused them to waiver or reconsider whether Jesus was the promised Messiah. They voted to crucify Him.

Joe and Nic stayed in the shadows until after Jesus was crucified. God used something in the passion of Jesus, however, to give them courage to trust again and come out of those shadows of fearing academic scorn.

Have you given thought to how you will represent your faith and Savior in the face of academic critique?

If not, why?

If so, describe how you are preparing to give a defense for the hope that is in you.

Reflection

Looking back over Mark 15, you see that hatred for Jesus seemed to come from all corners: politicians, soldiers, religious leaders, criminals, commoners, and academics.

If you read the following passages, you will discover it is not paranoia but prudence that should make you want to prepare to defend your faith and practice.

In **2 Timothy 3:12** and **John 15:18-20**, what persecutions are promised the saints? Why?

In **John 17:14-15**, what did Jesus pray regarding persecution of the saints?

In **Matthew 10:22** and **5:11-12**, what promises did Jesus make to saints who are persecuted?

Walking in Jesus' Footsteps Immediately

Another important thing to notice from Jesus' examples in Mark 15 is the ongoing redemptive work of God. In this chapter a criminal gave his life to Jesus, a centurion confessed Christ as the Son of God, and two academics stepped into God's light.

Not immediately recognizing or appreciating Jesus is not necessarily a terminal event. Just look at the hundreds or thousands who threw Jesus out of the county in Mark 5 and flocked to Him later in Mark 6 on the testimony of what the Lord had done for one man and the loving mercy God had had on that man.

Who have you encountered that rejected your testimony about Jesus, or persecuted you for your faith?

What will you do to continue trying to be a redemptive ambassador of reconciliation toward them?

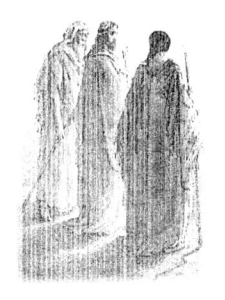

Mark 16

Go Forth In The Promises And Power Of God

Mapping the Path Forward

This concluding chapter of Mark's Gospel is so very hopeful and encouraging! Bask in its profound brevity. Take comfort in the promises of power it holds for you as God's servant to humanity through Christian healthcare.

What does this chapter have to say to you?

- God understands your very busy schedule. He has given you the wisdom and resources to minister even through busy periods.

- You never need to feel alone in serving God through healthcare. God is with you always.

- You don't have to fall into the trap of thinking you must provide Christian healthcare in your own wisdom and power. You serve daily in Christ's wisdom and power.

- Being guided by God's principles is always an honorable way of conduct.

- God's got you completely covered: the Holy Spirit indwells you and Jesus intercedes for you from heaven.

Plan for Delays
(Mark 16:1-8)

16 ¹When the Sabbath was over, Mary Magdalene, Mary the mother of James, and Salome bought spices, so they could go and anoint Him. ² Very early in the morning, on the first day of the week, they went to the tomb at sunrise. ³ They were saying to one another, "Who will roll away the stone from the entrance to the tomb for us?" ⁴ Looking up, they observed that the stone—which was very large—had been rolled away. ⁵ When they entered the tomb, they saw a young man dressed in a long white robe sitting on the right side; they were amazed and alarmed.

⁶ "Don't be alarmed," he told them. "You are looking for Jesus the Nazarene, who was crucified. He has been resurrected! He is not here! See the place where they put Him. ⁷ But go, tell His disciples and Peter, 'He is going ahead of you to Galilee; you will see Him there just as He told you.'"

⁸ So they went out and started running from the tomb, because trembling and astonishment overwhelmed them. And they said nothing to anyone, since they were afraid.

You can't always do what you want to do when you want to do it. Because of the Jewish laws and customs surrounding the Passover and the Sabbath, the women couldn't anoint Jesus at His burial. There was a delay that couldn't be helped. Yet they had a plan. They came back to finish their work at the first opportunity.

Under the pressure of workday constraints and schedules, you may not always get a chance to finish a conversation, teach a soul, or pray for a patient as you feel called to do. If this happens occasionally, you might get annoyed or feel bad. If this happens frequently, you may either develop a sense of guilt or even worse, stop caring about your patients' spiritual concerns.

Have a plan for such situations (and add your own ideas):

- Make an after-hours phone call.

- Send a card.

- Schedule a follow-up visit. (A workman is worth his wages. You can chart the ICD-9 code V62.89 or ICD-10 code Z65.8 for counseling or referring a patient having a spiritual struggle.)

- Use your referral network.

-

-

If God is leading you to speak light, truth, and hope to someone, pray for God's wisdom on how to obey Him and serve your patient. Take heart and be bold: if God is leading you, He'll go before you and make provision.

Are You Expecting Him to Appear?
(Mark 16:5-13)

⁵ When they entered the tomb, they saw a young man dressed in a long white robe sitting on the right side; they were amazed and alarmed.

⁶ "Don't be alarmed," he told them. "You are looking for Jesus the Nazarene, who was crucified. He has been resurrected! He is not here! See the place where they put Him. ⁷ But go, tell His disciples and Peter, 'He is going ahead of you to Galilee; you will see Him there just as He told you.'"

⁸ So they went out and started running from the tomb, because trembling and astonishment overwhelmed them. And they said nothing to anyone, since they were afraid.

⁹ Early on the first day of the week, after He had risen, He appeared first to Mary Magdalene, out of whom He had driven seven demons. ¹⁰ She went and reported to those who had been with Him, as they were mourning and weeping. ¹¹ Yet, when they heard that He was alive and had been seen by her, they did not believe it. ¹² Then after this, He appeared in a different form to two of them walking on their way into the country. ¹³ And they went and reported it to the rest, who did not believe them either.

Let's grant that nobody had ever seen a resurrection before, so Jesus returning alive from the dead in a glorified, incurruptible, immortal body was a completely alien idea. Not expecting to see Him was understandable.

However, you don't have such an excuse for not expecting to see God in your practice (see 1 Corinthians 15:1-11). In addition, as believers, you are indwelled by the Holy Spirit (John 14:15-26). Jesus is already with you!

Therefore, you can never enter into a patient, peer, family, or coworker encounter and legitimately whisper to yourself, "I hope God shows up." Your whispered prayer should instead be something like:

Lord you promised to give me wisdom if I ask, so I'm asking.
(James 1:5-8)

You promised to remind me of the things you've said and give me the words I need in times of trial, so I'm listening for them.
(John 14:26 and Mark 13:11)

You've said that as your ambassador of reconciliation, I go through this world in your authority.
(2 Corinthians 5:20; Ephesians 6:20 and Matthew 28:18-20)

You've promised you will never leave or forsake me.
(Deuteronomy 31:6 and Hebrews 13:5)

So, 'Here I am. Send me.'
(Isaiah 6:8)

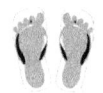

Principles, Practices, and Preferences
(Mark 16:14-18)

¹⁴ Later, He appeared to the Eleven themselves as they were reclining at the table. He rebuked their unbelief and hardness of heart, because they did not believe those who saw Him after He had been resurrected. ¹⁵ Then He said to them, "Go into all the world and preach the gospel to the whole creation. ¹⁶ Whoever believes and is baptized will be saved, but whoever does not believe will be condemned. ¹⁷ And these signs will accompany those who believe: In My name they will drive out demons; they will speak in new languages; ¹⁸ they will pick up snakes; if they should drink anything deadly, it will never harm them; they will lay hands on the sick, and they will get well."

Certainly this passage is one that stirs controversy among believers and denominations. It is not the purpose or presumption here to settle all the issues it raises. Rather, based upon Jesus' own prayer for you (John 17:20-23), presume that the principles, if not the specific practices or preferences, listed in this passage still apply to you.

First, the whole world should hear the Good News of Jesus. You are the beautiful feet that can bring that Good News (Romans 10:14-17).

Second, whoever believes in the person and work of Jesus will be saved (John 3:14-18; Romans 10:8-13).

Third, baptism was and remains an outward sign and public profession of an inner event of repentance, trusting Jesus, being born again, and being made alive in spirit by the indwelling of God's Holy Spirit. Getting wet, one way or another, isn't the act that saves. It is not likely something you will do in your routine practice, nor do you need to.

Fourth, Scripture is clear that some believers manifested remarkable spiritual gifts. They were given these signs to authenticate their message. There is nothing in Scripture to say that God will not continue to give those signs to those who need them. However, the need for them – in your contemporary context – has been reduced by the existence of other signs, such as the global number of believers, the existence of the church despite severe persecution, God's written Word, and the gracious, selfless, charitable acts of Jesus' followers worldwide and locally.

If it is necessary, in God's view, that you manifest a sign to convince someone, He will do it. However, first be an excellent healthcare practitioner, which wins you an audience of trust and respect. Tell your story of what the Lord has done for you and the loving mercy He's had on you. Then, as the appropriate opportunity presents itself, share the Good News of Jesus. You may well get to see the greatest miracle of all take place in the heart of your audience.

Jesus Is Interceding for You
(Mark 16:19-20)

19 Then after speaking to them, the Lord Jesus was taken up into heaven and sat down at the right hand of God. 20 And they went out and preached everywhere, the Lord working with them and confirming the word by the accompanying signs.

If you still wonder if God will enter into your Christian healthcare practice with power, according to His promises, read **Romans 8:31-39** and **Hebrews 7:22-26**.

What is God speaking to you through these texts?

Reflection

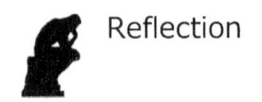

Which module in this study gave you the most encouragement? Why?

What aspect or feature of the topics introduced do you desire God to manifest more fully in your life and practice?

Pray now and ask Him for those things. Persist in that prayer until He answers. Record how He answered your prayer.

Walking in Jesus' Footsteps Immediately

Most Christians in healthcare are so busy during their shift that they don't pause to pray and invite God to be a part of each interaction. If you want to welcome God into your practice, you may be better off to pray an umbrella request prior to the start of your shift.

Craft a prayer in your own words that acknowledges God is for you and for your patients, that He wants you to be His witness by exposing Jesus, that He wants you to exude His love, wisdom, and power, and that you want to be His faithful servant today.

Appendix I

A Harmony of the Gospels, by A.T. Robertson

Outline courtesy of the Project Gutenberg Online eBook accessed 11 May 2015.

The Analytical Outline of the Harmony is available at:
http://www.gutenberg.org/files/36264/36264-h/36264-h.htm - outline

AN OUTLINE OF THE HARMONY

THE SOURCES OF THE GOSPELS

In The Dedication Luke Explains His Method Of Research
Luke 1:1-4.

THE PRE-EXISTENT STATE OF CHRIST AND HIS INCARNATION

In His Introduction John Pictures Christ
As The Word (Logos)
John 1:1-18.

THE TWO GENEALOGIES IN MATTHEW AND LUKE

Apparently Joseph's Genealogy In Matthew
And Mary's In Luke
Matt. 1:1-17; Luke 3:23-38.

THE BIRTH AND CHILDHOOD OF THE BAPTIST AND OF JESUS

The Annunciation Of The Birth
Of The Baptist To Zacharias
Luke 1:5-25.

The Annunciation To The Virgin Mary
Of The Birth Of Jesus
Luke 1:26-38.

The Song Of Elizabeth To Mary Upon Her Visit
Luke 1:39-45.

The Magnificat Of Mary
Luke 1:46-56.

The Birth And Childhood Of The Baptist
And His Desert Life
Luke 1:57-80.

The Annunciation To Joseph Of The Birth Of Jesus
Matt. 1:18-25.

The Birth Of Jesus
Luke 2:1-7.

The Praise Of The Angels And
The Homage Of The Shepherds
Luke 2:8-20.

The Circumcision Of Jesus
Luke 2:21.

The Presentation In The Temple With
The Homage Of Simeon And Anna
Luke 2:22-38.

Magi Visit The New-Born King Of The Jews
Matt. 2:1-12.

The Child Jesus Carried To Egypt,
And The Children At Bethlehem Slain
Matt. 2:13-18.

The Child Brought From Egypt To Nazareth
Matt. 2:19-23; Luke 2:39.

The Childhood Of Jesus At Nazareth
Luke 2:40.

The Visit Of The Boy Jesus To Jerusalem
When Twelve Years Old
Luke 2:41-50.

The Eighteen Years At Nazareth
Luke 2:51-52.

THE BEGINNING OF THE BAPTIST'S MINISTRY

The Time Of The Beginning
Mark 1:1; Luke 3:1-2.

The Message And The Messenger
Mark 1:2-6; Matt. 3:1-6; Luke 3:3-6.

A Specimen Of John's Preaching
Matt. 3:7-10; Luke 3:7-14.

The Forerunner's Picture Of The Messiah
Before Seeing Him
Mark 1:7-8; Matt. 3:11-12; Luke 3:15-18.

THE BEGINNING OF CHRIST'S PUBLIC MINISTRY

Jesus Baptized By John In The Jordan
Mark 1:9-11; Matt. 3:13-17; Luke 3:21-23.

The Three Temptations Of Jesus
Mark 1:12-13; Matt. 4:1-11; Luke 4:1-13.

The Testimony Of The Baptist
To The Committee Of The Sanhedrin
John 1:19-28.

John's Identification Of Jesus As The Messiah
John 1:29-34.

Jesus Makes His First Disciples

John 1:35-51.

Jesus Works His First Miracle
John 2:1-11.

Jesus Makes A First Sojourn At Capernaum,
Accompanied By His Kindred And His Early Disciples
John 2:12.

The First Cleansing Of The Temple At The Passover
John 2:13-22.

The Interview Of Nicodemus With Jesus
John 2:23-3:21.

The Parallel Ministry Of Jesus And
John With John's Loyalty To Jesus
John 3:22-36.

Christ's Reasons For Leaving Judea
Mark 1:14; Matt. 4:12; Luke 3:19-20; 4:14; John 4:1-4.

Jesus In Samaria At Jacob's Well And In Sychar
John 4:5-42.

The Arrival Of Jesus In Galilee
John 4:43-45.

THE GREAT GALILEAN MINISTRY

Eight Groups in the Period

The Rejection at Nazareth and the New Home in Capernaum

The First Tour of Galilee with the Four Fishermen and the Call of Matthew (Levi) on the Return with the Growing Fame of Jesus

The Sabbath Controversy in Jerusalem and in Galilee

The Choice of the Twelve and the Sermon on the Mount

The Spread of Christ's Influence and the Inquiry from John in Prison

The Second Tour of Galilee (now with the Twelve) and the Intense Hostility of the Pharisees

The First Great Group of Parables with the Visit to Gerasa (Khersa) and to Nazareth (final one)

The Third Tour of Galilee (following the Twelve) and the Effect on Herod Antipas

General Account Of His Teaching In Galilee
Mark 1:14-15; Matt. 4:17; Luke 4:14-15.

The Healing At Cana Of The Son
Of A Courtier Of Capernaum
John 4:46-54.

The First Rejection At Nazareth
Luke 4:16-31.

The New Home In Capernaum
Matt. 4:13-16.

Jesus Finds Four Fishers Of Men In Four Fishermen
Mark 1:16-20; Matt. 4:18-22; Luke 5:1-11.

The Excitement In The Synagogue Because Of The
Teaching Of Jesus And The Healing Of
A Demoniac On The Sabbath
Mark 1:21-28; Luke 4:31-37.

He Heals Peter's Mother-In-Law And Many Others
Mark 1:29-34; Matt. 8:14-17; Luke 4:38-41.

The First Tour Of Galilee With The Four Fishermen
Mark 1:35-39; Matt. 4:23-25; Luke 4:42-44.

A Leper Healed And Much Popular Excitement
Mark 1:40-45; Matt. 8:2-4; Luke 5:12-16.

Thronged In Capernaum, He Heals A Paralytic Lowered
Through The Roof Of Peter's House
Mark 2:1-12; Matt. 9:1-8; Luke 5:17-26.

The Call Of Matthew (Levi) And
His Reception In Honor Of Jesus
Mark 2:13-17; Matt. 9:9-13; Luke 5:27-32.

Jesus In Three Parables Defends His Disciples For
Feasting Instead Of Fasting
Mark 2:18-22; Matt. 9:14-17; Luke 5:33-39.

At A Feast In Jerusalem (Possibly The Passover) Jesus
Heals A Lame Man On The Sabbath And Defends This
Action To The Pharisees In A Great Discourse
John 5:1-47.

Another Sabbath Controversy With The Pharisees When
The Disciples Pluck Ears Of Grain In The Fields
Mark 2:23-28; Matt. 12:1-8; Luke 6:1-5.

A Third Sabbath Controversy With The Pharisees
Over The Healing Of A Man With A Withered Hand
In A Synagogue
Mark 3:1-6; Matt. 12:9-14; Luke 6:6-11.

Jesus Teaches And Heals Great Multitudes
By The Sea Of Galilee
Mark 3:7-12; Matt. 12:15-21.

After A Night Of Prayer Jesus Selects Twelve Apostles
Mark 3:13-19; Luke 6:12-16.

The Sermon On The Mount. Privileges And
Requirements Of The Messianic Reign,
Christ's Standard Of Righteousness
Matt. 5-7; Luke 6:17-49.

   The Place and the Audience
   Matt. 5:1-2; Luke 6:17-19.

   (1) The Introduction: The Beatitudes and the Woes.
   Privileges of the Messiah's Subjects
    Matt. 5:3-12; Luke 6:20-26.

   (2) The Theme of the Sermon: Christ's Standard of
   Righteousness in Contrast with that of the Scribes and
   Pharisees
    Matt. 5:13-20.

   (3) Christ's Ethical Teaching Superior to that of the Scribes
   (both the Old Testament and the Oral Law) in Six Items or
   Illustrations (Murder, Adultery, Divorce, Oaths,
   Retaliations, Love of Enemies)
    Matt. 5:21-48; Luke 6:27-30, 32-36.

   (4) The Practice of Real Righteousness unlike the
   Ostentatious Hypocrisy of the Pharisees as in
   Almsgiving, Prayer, Fasting
    Matt. 6:1-18.

(5) Single-hearted Devotion to God as Opposed to
Worldly Aims and Anxieties
 Matt. 6:19-34.

(6) Captious Criticism, or Judging Others
 Matt. 7:1-6; Luke 6:37-42.

(7) Prayer and the Golden Rule
 Matt. 7:7-12; Luke 6:31.

(8) The Conclusion of the Sermon. The Lesson of Personal
Righteousness Driven Home by Powerful Parables
 Matt. 7:13-8:1; Luke 6:43-49.

Jesus Heals A Centurion's Servant At Capernaum
Matt. 8:5-13; Luke 7:1-10.

He Raises A Widow's Son At Nain
Luke 7:11-17.

The Message From The Baptist And The Eulogy Of Jesus
Matt. 11:2-19; Luke 7:18-35.

Woes Upon The Cities Of Opportunity. The Claims Of
Christ As The Teacher About The Father
Matt. 11:20-30.

The Anointing Of Christ's Feet By A Sinful Woman
In The House Of Simon A Pharisee.
The Parable Of The Two Debtors
Luke 7:36-50.

The Second Tour Of Galilee
Luke 8:1-3.

Blasphemous Accusation Of League With Beelzebub
Mark 3:19-30; Matt. 12:22-37.

Scribes And Pharisees Demand A Sign
Matt. 12:38-45.

Christ's Mother And Brethren Seek To Take Him Home
Mark 3:31-35; Matt. 12:46-50; Luke 8:19-21.

The First Great Group Of Parables
Mark 4:1-34; Matt. 13:1-53; Luke 8:4-18.

  Introduction to the Group
  Mark 4:1-2; Matt. 13:1-3; Luke 8:4.

  1: *To the Crowds by the Sea*

  (a) Parable of the Sower
  Mark 4:3-25; Matt. 13:3-23; Luke 8:5-18.

  (b) Parable of the Seed Growing of Itself
  Mark 4:26-29.

(c) Parable of the Tares
Matt. 13:24-30.

(d) Parable of the Mustard Seed
Mark 4:30-32; Matt. 13:31-32.

(e) Parable of the Leaven and Many Such Parables
Mark 4:33-34; Matt. 13:33-35.

2. *To the Disciples in the House*

(a) Explanation of the Parable of the Tares

Matt. 13:36-43.

(b) The Parable of the Hid Treasure
Matt. 13:44.

(c) The Parable of the Pearl of Great Price
Matt. 13:45-46.

(d) The Parable of the Net
Matt. 13:47-50.

(e) The Parable of the Householder
Matt. 13:51-53.

In Crossing The Lake, Jesus Stills The Tempest
Mark 4:35-41; Matt. 8:18, 23-27; Luke 8:22-25.

Beyond The Lake Jesus Heals The Gerasene Demoniac
Mark 5:1-20; Matt. 8:28-34; Luke 8:26-39.

The Return And The Healing Of Jairus' Daughter And Of The Woman Who Only Touched Christ's Garment
Mark 5:21-43; Matt. 9:18-26; Luke 8:40-56.

He Heals Two Blind Men And A Dumb Demoniac, A Blasphemous Accusation
Matt. 9:27-34.

The Last Visit To Nazareth
Mark 6:1-6; Matt. 13:54-58.

The Third Tour Of Galilee After Instructing The Twelve And Sending Them Forth By Twos
Mark 6:6-13; Matt. 9:35-11:1; Luke 9:1-6.

The Guilty Fears Of Herod Antipas In Tiberias About Jesus Because He Had Beheaded The Baptist In Machærus
Mark 6:14-29; Matt. 14:1-12; Luke 9:7-9.

THE SPECIAL TRAINING OF THE TWELVE IN DISTRICTS AROUND GALILEE

The First Retirement. The Twelve Return, And Jesus Retires With Them Beyond The Lake To Rest. Feeding Of The Five Thousand
Mark 6:30-44; Matt. 14:13-21; Luke 9:10-17; John 6:1-13.

The Prevention Of The Revolutionary Purpose To
Proclaim Jesus King (A Political Messiah)
Mark 6:45-46; Matt. 14:22-23; John 6:14-15.

The Peril To The Twelve In The Storm At Sea And
Christ's Coming To Them On The Water In The Darkness
Mark 6:47-52; Matt. 14:24-33; John 6:16-21.

The Reception At Gennesaret
Mark 6:53-56; Matt. 14:34-36.

The Collapse Of The Galilean Campaign Because Jesus
Will Not Conform To Popular Messianic Expectations
John 6:22-71.

Pharisees From Jerusalem Reproach Jesus For
Allowing His Disciples To Disregard Their Traditions
About Ceremonial Defilement Of The Hands.
A Puzzling Parable In Reply
Mark 7:1-23; Matt. 15:1-20; John 7:1.

The Second Withdrawal To The Region
Of Tyre And Sidon And The Healing Of
The Daughter Of A Syro-Phoenician Woman
Mark 7:24-30; Matt. 15:21-28.

The Third Withdrawal North Through Phoenicia And
East Towards Hermon And South Into Decapolis
(Keeping Out Of The Territory Of Herod Antipas) With
The Healing Of The Deaf And Dumb Man And The
Feeding Of The Four Thousand
Mark 7:31-8:9; Matt. 15:29-38.

The Brief Visit To Magadan (Dalmanutha) In Galilee And
The Sharp Attack By The Pharisees And Sadducees.
(Note Their Appearance Now Against Jesus)
Mark 8:10-12; Matt. 15:39-16:4.

The Fourth Retirement To Bethsaida Julias In The
Tetrarchy Of Herod Philip With Sharp Rebuke Of
The Dullness Of The Disciples On The Way Across
And The Healing Of A Blind Man In Bethsaida
Mark 8:13-26; Matt. 16:5-12.

Near Cæsarea Philippi Jesus Tests The Faith
Of The Twelve In His Messiahship
Mark 8:27-30; Matt. 16:13-20; Luke 9:18-21.

Jesus Distinctly Foretells That He, The Messiah, Will Be
Rejected And Killed And Will Rise The Third Day
Mark 8:31-37; Matt. 16:21-26; Luke 9:22-25.

The Coming Of The Son Of Man In That Generation
Mark 8:38-9:1; Matt. 16:27-28; Luke 9:26-27.

The Transfiguration Of Jesus On A Mountain
(Probably Hermon) Near Cæsarea Philippi
Mark 9:2-8; Matt. 17:1-8; Luke 9:28-36.

The Puzzle Of The Three Disciples About The
Resurrection And About Elijah On Their
Way Down The Mountain
Mark 9:9-13; Matt. 17:9-13; Luke 9:36.

The Demoniac Boy, Whom The Disciples Could Not Heal
Mark 9:14-29; Matt. 17:14-20; Luke 9:37-43.

Returning Privately Through Galilee,
He Again Foretells His Death And Resurrection
Mark 9:30-32; Matt. 17:22-23; Luke 9:43-45.

Jesus, The Messiah, Pays The Half-Shekel For The Temple
Matt. 17:24-27.

The Twelve Contend As To Who Shall Be
The Greatest Under The Messiah's Reign.
His Subjects Must Be Childlike
Mark 9:33-37; Matt. 18:1-5; Luke 9:46-48.

The Mistaken Zeal Of The Apostle John Rebuked By Jesus
In Pertinent Parables
Mark 9:38-50; Matt. 18:6-14; Luke 9:49-50.

Right Treatment Of A Brother Who Has Sinned Against
One, And Duty Of Patiently Forgiving A Brother
(Parable Of The Unmerciful Servant)
Matt. 18:15-35.

The Messiah's Followers Must Give Up Everything
For His Service
Matt. 8:19-22; Luke 9:57-62.

The Unbelieving Brothers Of Jesus Counsel Him To
Exhibit Himself In Judea, And He Rejects The Advice
John 7:2-9.

He Goes Privately To Jerusalem Through Samaria
Luke 9:51-56; John 7:10.

THE LATER JUDEAN MINISTRY

The Coming Of Jesus To The Feast Of Tabernacles Creates
Intense Excitement Concerning The Messiahship
John 7:11-52.

Story Of An Adulterous Woman Brought
To Jesus For Judgment
John 7:53-8:11.

After The Feast Of Tabernacles In The Temple
Jesus Angers The Pharisees By Claiming
To Be The Light Of The World
John 8:12-20.

The Pharisees Attempt To Stone Jesus
When He Exposes Their Sinfulness
John 8:21-59.

Jesus Heals A Man Born Blind Who Outwits The
Pharisees. The Rulers Forbid The Recognition Of Jesus As
The Messiah. The Conversion Of The Healed Man
John 9:1-41.

In The Parable (Allegory) Of The Good Shepherd
Jesus Draws The Picture Of The Hostile Pharisees
And Intimates That He Is Going To Die For His Flock
And Come To Life Again
John 10:1-21.

The Mission Of The Seventy.
Christ's Joy In Their Work On Their Return
Luke 10:1-24.

Jesus Answers A Lawyer's Question As To Eternal Life,
Giving The Parable Of The Good Samaritan
Luke 10:25-37.

Jesus The Guest Of Martha And Mary
Luke 10:38-42.

Jesus Again Gives A Model Of Prayer
And Encourages His Disciples To Pray.
Parable Of The Importunate Friend
Luke 11:1-13.

Blasphemous Accusation Of League With Beelzebub
Luke 11:14-36.

While Breakfasting With A Pharisee, Jesus Severely
Denounces The Pharisees And Lawyers
And Excites Their Enmity
Luke 11:37-54.

He Speaks To His Disciples And A Vast Throng About
Hypocrisy, Covetousness (Parable Of The Rich Fool),
Worldly Anxieties, Watchfulness (Parable Of The
Waiting Servants And Of The Wise Steward),
And His Own Approaching Passion
Luke 12.

All Must Repent Or Perish. (Two Current Tragedies);
Parable Of The Barren Fig Tree
Luke 13:1-9.

Jesus Heals A Crippled Woman On The Sabbath And
Defends Himself Against The Ruler Of The Synagogue.
Repetition Of The Parables Of The Mustard Seed
And Of The Leaven
Luke 13:10-21.

At The Feast Of Dedication Jesus Will Not Yet Openly Say
That He Is The Messiah. The Jews Try To Stone Him
John 10:22-39.

THE LATER PEREAN MINISTRY

The Withdrawal From Jerusalem
To Bethany Beyond Jordan
John 10:40-42.

Teaching In Perea, On A Journey Toward Jerusalem,
Warned Against Herod Antipas
Luke 13:22-35.

While Dining (Breakfasting) With A Chief Pharisee,
He Again Heals On The Sabbath And Defends Himself.
Three Parables Suggested By The Occasion
Luke 14:1-24.

Great Crowds Follow Him, And He Warns Them To
Count The Cost Of Discipleship To Him
Luke 14:25-35.

The Pharisees And The Scribes Murmur Against Jesus For
Receiving Sinners. He Defends Himself By Three Great
Parables (The Lost Sheep, The Lost Coin, The Lost Son)
Luke 15:1-32.

Three Parables On Stewardship (To The Disciples,
The Parable Of The Unjust Steward; To The Pharisees,
The Parable Of The Rich Man And Lazarus; To The
Disciples, The Parable Of The Unprofitable Servants)
Luke 16:1-17:10.

Jesus Raises Lazarus From The Dead
John 11:1-44.

The Effect Of The Raising Of Lazarus (On The People,
On The Sanhedrin, On The Movements Of Jesus)
John 11:45-54.

Jesus Starts On The Last Journey To Jerusalem
By Way Of Samaria And Galilee
Luke 17:11-37.

Two Parables On Prayer (The Importunate Widow,
The Pharisee And The Publican)
Luke 18:1-14.

Going From Galilee Through Perea, He Teaches
Concerning Divorce
Mark 10:1-12; Matt. 19:1-12.

Christ And Children And The Failure Of The Disciples
To Understand The Attitude Of Jesus
Mark 10:13-16; Matt. 19:13-15; Luke 18:15-17.

The Rich Young Ruler, The Perils Of Riches, And
Amazement Of The Disciples. The Rewards Of Forsaking
All To Follow The Messiah Will Be Great, But Will Be
Sovereign (Parable Of The Laborers In The Vineyard)
Mark 10:17-31; Matt. 19:16-20:16; Luke 18:18-30.

Jesus Again Foretells To The Disciples His Death And
Resurrection, And Rebukes The Selfish Ambition Of
James And John
Mark 10:32-45; Matt. 20:17-28; Luke 18:31-34.

Blind Bartimæus And His Companion Healed
Mark 10:46-52; Matt. 20:29-34; Luke 18:35-43.

Jesus Visits Zacchæus, And Speaks The Parable
Of The Pounds, And Sets Out For Jerusalem
Luke 19:1-28.

THE LAST PUBLIC MINISTRY IN JERUSALEM

Jesus Arrives At Bethany Near Jerusalem
John 11:55 12:1, 9-11.

His Triumphal Entry Into Jerusalem As The Messiah
Mark 11:1-11; Matt. 21:1-11, 14-17; Luke 19:29-44;
John 12:12-19.

The Barren Fig Tree Cursed, And The Second Cleansing Of The Temple
Mark 11:12-18; Matt. 21:18-19, 12-13; Luke 19:45-48.

The Desire Of Some Greeks To See Jesus Puzzles The Disciples And Leads Jesus In Agitation Of Soul To Interpret Life And Death As Sacrifice And To Show How By Being "Lifted Up" He Will Draw All Men To Him
John 12:20-50.

The Barren Fig Tree Found To Have Withered
Mark 11:19-25; Matt. 21:19-22; Luke 21:37-38.

The Rulers (Sanhedrin) Formally Challenge The Authority Of Jesus As An Accredited Teacher (Rabbi)
Mark 11:27-12:12; Matt. 21:23-22:14; Luke 20:1-19.

The Pharisees And The Herodians Try To Ensnare Jesus About Paying Tribute To Cæsar
Mark 12:13-17; Matt. 22:15-22; Luke 20:20-26.

The Sadducees Ask Him A Puzzling Question About The Resurrection
Mark 12:18-27; Matt. 22:23-33; Luke 20:27-40.

The Pharisees Rejoice Over The Rout Of The Sadducees And A Pharisaic Lawyer Asks Jesus A Legal Question
Mark 12:28-34; Matt. 22:34-40.

Jesus, To The Joy Of The Multitude, Silences His Enemies
By The Pertinent Question Of The Messiah's Descent
From David And Lordship Over David
Mark 12:35-37; Matt. 22:41-46; Luke 20:41-44.

In His Last Public Discourse, Jesus Solemnly Denounces
The Scribes And Pharisees
Mark 12:38-40; Matt. 23:1-39; Luke 20:45-47.

Jesus Closely Observes The Contributions In The Temple,
And Commends The Poor Widow's Gift
Mark 12:41-44; Luke 21:1-4.

IN THE SHADOW WITH JESUS

Sitting On The Mount Of Olives, Jesus Speaks To His
Disciples About The Destruction Of Jerusalem, And His
Own Second Coming In Apocalyptic Language.
The Great Eschatological Discourse
Mark 13:1-37; Matt. 24, 25; Luke 21:5-36.

Jesus Predicts His Crucifixion Two Days Hence
(Jewish Friday)
Mark 14:1-2; Matt. 26:1-5; Luke 22:1-2.

At The Feast In The House Of Simon The Leper
Mary Of Bethany Anoints Jesus For His Burial
Mark 14:3-9; Matt. 26:6-13; John 12:2-8.

Judas, Stung By The Rebuke Of Jesus At The Feast,
Bargains With The Rulers To Betray Jesus
Mark 14:10-11; Matt. 26:14-16; Luke 22:3-6.

The Preparation For The Paschal Meal At The Home Of A
Friend (Possibly That Of John Mark's Father And Mother)
Mark 14:12-16; Matt. 26:17-19; Luke 22:7-13.

Jesus Partakes Of The Paschal Meal With The Twelve
Apostles And Rebukes Their Jealousy
Mark 14:17; Matt. 26:20; Luke 22:14-16, 24-30.

During The Paschal Meal, Jesus Washes
The Feet Of His Disciples
John 13:1-20.

At The Paschal Meal Jesus Points Out
Judas As The Betrayer
Mark 14:18-21; Matt. 26:21-25; Luke 22:21-23;
John 13:21-30.

After The Departure Of Judas Jesus Warns The Disciples
(Peter In Particular) Against Desertion, While All
Protest Their Loyalty
Mark 14:27-31; Matt. 26:31-35; Luke 22:31-38;
John 13:31-38.

Jesus Institutes The Memorial Of Eating Bread And
Drinking Wine
Mark 14:22-25; Matt. 26:26-29; Luke 22:17-20;
1 Cor. 11:23-26.

The Farewell Discourse To His Disciples
In The Upper Room
John 14.

The Discourse On The Way To Gethsemane
John 15, 16.

Christ's Intercessory Prayer
John 17.

Going Forth To Gethsemane, Jesus Suffers Long In Agony
Mark 14:26, 32-42; Matt. 26:30, 36-46; Luke 22:39-46;
John 18:1.

THE ARREST, TRIAL, CRUCIFIXION, AND BURIAL OF JESUS

Jesus Is Betrayed, Arrested, And Forsaken
Mark 14:43-52; Matt. 26:47-56; Luke 22:47-53; John 18:2-12.

Jesus First Examined By Annas, The Ex-High Priest
John 18:12-14, 19-23.

Jesus Hurriedly Tried And Condemned By Caiaphas And The Sanhedrin, Who Mock And Buffet Him
Mark 14:53, 55-65; Matt. 26:57, 59-68; Luke 22:54, 63-65; John 18:24.

Peter Thrice Denies His Lord
Mark 14:54, 66-72; Matt. 26:58, 69-75; Luke 22:54-62; John 18:15-18, 25-27.

After Dawn, Jesus Is Formally Condemned By The Sanhedrin
Mark 15:1; Matt. 27:1; Luke 22:66-71.

Remorse And Suicide Of Judas The Betrayer
Matt. 27:3-10; Acts 1:18-19.

Jesus Before Pilate The First Time
Mark 15:1-5; Matt. 27:2, 11-14; Luke 23:1-5; John 18:28-38.

Jesus Before Herod Antipas The Tetrarch
Luke 23:6-12.

Jesus The Second Time Before Pilate
Mark 15:6-15; Matt. 27:15-26; Luke 23:13-25; John 18:39-19:16.

The Roman Soldiers Mock Jesus
Mark 15:16-19; Matt. 27:27-30.

Jesus On The Way To The Cross (Via Dolorosa)
On Golgotha
Mark 15:20-23; Matt. 27:31-34; Luke 23:26-33;
John 19:16-17.

The First Three Hours On The Cross
Mark 15:24-32; Matt. 27:35-44; Luke 23:33-43;
John 19:18-27.

The Three Hours Of Darkness From Noon To Three P.M.
Mark 15:33-37; Matt. 27:45-50; Luke 23:44-46;
John 19:28-30.

The Phenomena Accompanying The Death Of Christ
Mark 15:38-41; Matt. 27:51-56; Luke 23:45, 47-49.

The Burial Of The Body Of Jesus In The Tomb Of
Joseph Of Arimathea After Proof Of His Death
Mark 15:42-46; Matt. 27:57-60; Luke 23:50-54;
John 19:31-42.

The Watch Of The Women By The Tomb Of Jesus
Mark 15:47; Matt. 27:61-66; Luke 23:55-56.

THE RESURRECTION, APPEARANCES, AND ASCENSION OF CHRIST

The Visit Of The Women To The Tomb Of Jesus
Mark 16:1; Matt. 28:1.

The Earthquake, The Rolling Away Of The Stone By An Angel, And The Fright Of The Roman Watchers
Matt. 28:2-4.

The Visit Of The Women To The Tomb Of Jesus About Sunrise Sunday Morning And The Message Of The Angels About The Empty Tomb
Mark 16:2-8; Matt. 28:5-8; Luke 24:1-8; John 20:1.

Mary Magdalene And The Other Women Report To The Apostles, And Peter And John Visit The Empty Tomb
Luke 24:9-12; John 20:2-10.

The Appearance Of Jesus To Mary Magdalene And The Message To The Disciples
Mark 16:9-11; John 20:11-18.

The Appearance Of Jesus To The Other Women
Matt. 28:9-10.

Some Of The Guard Report To The Jewish Rulers
Matt. 28:11-15.

The Appearance To Two Disciples (Cleopas And Another) On The Way To Emmaus
Mark 16:12-13; Luke 24:13-32.

The Report Of The Two Disciples And
The News Of The Appearance To Simon Peter
Luke 24:33-35; 1 Cor. 15:5.

The Appearance To The Astonished Disciples
(Thomas Absent) With A Commission And
Their Failure To Convince Thomas
Mark 16:14; Luke 24:36-43; John 20:19-25.

The Appearance To The Disciples The Next Sunday Night
And The Convincing Of Thomas
John 20:26-31; 1 Cor. 15:5.

The Appearance To Seven Disciples Beside The Sea Of
Galilee. The Miraculous Draught Of Fishes
John 21.

The Appearance To About Five Hundred
On An Appointed Mountain In Galilee,
And A Commission Given
Mark 16:15-18; Matt. 28:16-20; 1 Cor. 15:6.

The Appearance To James The Brother Of Jesus
1 Cor. 15:7.

The Appearance To The Disciples With
Another Commission
Luke 24:44-49; Acts 1:3-8.

The Last Appearance And The Ascension
Mark 16:19-20; Luke 24:50-53; Acts 1:9-12.

CPSIA information can be obtained
at www.ICGtesting.com
Printed in the USA
FSOW03n1650101116
27241FS